DIVERTICULITIS COOKBOOK AFTER 60

OVER 2000 DAYS OF EASY, FLARE-UP PREVENTIVE RECIPES | FEATURING A 90-DAY MEAL PLAN, DAILY MENTAL HEALTH TIPS, AND SUPPLEMENT GUIDE

SHARON WILLIAMS

TABLE OF CONTENTS

Scan the QR Code and access your 3 bonuses in digital format

🔥 **Bonus 1: SUPPLEMENT GUIDE**

🔥 **Bonus 2: DAILY MENTAL HEALTH TIPS**

🔥 **Bonus 3: 90Day Meal Plan with Adjustments and Tips**

1

THE BASICS OF DIVERTICULITIS

What is Diverticulitis?

Diverticulitis is a digestive condition that primarily affects the large intestine, also known as the colon. It arises when small pouches, or diverticula, which can form along the walls of the colon, become inflamed or infected. These pouches usually form as a consequence of strain on weak areas in the colon, usually brought on by a low fiber diet and age-related changes in the colon's structure. While the formation of diverticula—known as diverticulosis—is relatively common and often symptom free, the situation escalates to diverticulitis when these pouches become inflamed.

Individuals above the age of 60 are more likely to have this illness. As the body ages, the colon's resilience decreases, which might contribute to the formation of diverticula and the subsequent risk of inflammation. This demographic shift is also influenced by lifetime dietary habits; older generations may not have consistently consumed the high fiber diets that help to prevent such conditions.

Diverticulitis can present with a range of symptoms, the most frequent of which is lower left abdominal discomfort, however it can also present with other symptoms as well. This pain can suddenly worsen and is often accompanied by other signs such as nausea, a marked change in bowel habits, fever, and, in severe cases, bleeding from the rectum. The discomfort and potential complications associated with diverticulitis significantly impact the quality of life, making it a serious concern for older adults who might already be managing other health issues.

Moreover, the factors that contribute to the development of diverticulitis include a diet low in fiber, which leads to harder stools and, consequently, more straining during bowel movements. This straining increases the pressure within the colon, which can lead to the formation of diverticula. Over time, if these pouches become blocked with fecal material, bacteria can build up and lead to infection or inflammation.

Preventive measures primarily revolve around dietary adjustments. Consuming more fiber rich meals, such as fruits, vegetables, and whole grains, can help produce softer stools and minimize strain during bowel movements, lowering the chance of pouch development. Moreover, staying hydrated by drinking plenty of fluids supports this process, as water helps to soften stool and promotes easier passage through the colon.

Management of the condition when symptoms do arise varies depending on the severity. Mild diverticulitis can sometimes be managed at home with a diet adjusted to enable the colon to heal, such as a clear liquid diet followed by a gradual reintroduction of solid meals. In more severe cases, treatment may involve antibiotics to clear the infection, and in rare instances where complications occur, surgery may be required to remove the affected portion of the colon.

Effectively diagnosing and treating diverticulitis is essential, particularly for people over 60, as prompt treatment can stop the illness from becoming worse and greatly reduce suffering. Awareness and education about this condition can empower individuals to make lifestyle choices that diminish the risk of its development and aid in maintaining a healthier, more comfortable life as they age.

Aging and Gut Health: Diverticulitis After 60

As we age, the body undergoes various changes, and the digestive system is no exception. One significant aspect of aging that affects gut health is the increased risk of conditions like diverticulitis, particularly after the age of 60. Understanding how aging impacts the gut and the specific risks and symptoms associated with diverticulitis is crucial for prevention and management.

The aging process naturally affects the structure and function of the digestive system. The strength and elasticity of the gastrointestinal (GI) tract's walls decrease, and the motility—how quickly and efficiently food moves through the digestive system—slows down. These changes can result in common age-related digestive issues such as constipation, increased gas, and bloating. For the large intestine, specifically, these changes can exacerbate the risk of developing diverticula—the small pouches that form in the colon wall, which are the hallmarks of diverticulosis.

When these diverticula become inflamed, the condition progresses to diverticulitis. The inflammation or infection of these pouches in older adults can be particularly severe due to the decreased efficiency of their immune systems. Additionally, as people age, their pain sensitivity may decrease, which means they might not notice or respond to the early warning signs of diverticulitis as quickly as younger individuals. This delay in discovery and treatment increases the likelihood of consequences, such as colon perforations or serious infections.

Symptoms of diverticulitis in the elderly may not present as typically as they do in younger individuals. While abdominal pain, fever, and changes in bowel habits are common symptoms across all ages, older adults might experience more subtle symptoms like mild abdominal tenderness or general malaise. This subtlety makes vigilance crucial for those caring for older adults or for the individuals themselves.

To mitigate these risks, there are several preventive measures that can be particularly beneficial for older adults:

Dietary Adjustments: A fiber rich diet is paramount. Fibers help to soften the stool and decrease transit time, alleviating pressure on the colon walls and reducing the likelihood of diverticula formation and inflammation. Fiber rich foods include whole grains, veggies, and fruits. However, older persons should gradually increase their fiber intake to avoid bloating and gas, which can be painful owing to reduced GI motility.

Adequate Hydration: With age, the sense of thirst might diminish, making dehydration a common issue among older adults. Ensuring adequate fluid intake helps soften the stool and promote easier bowel movements, reducing strain on the colon.

Regular Physical Activity: Regular, moderate exercise can help keep your digestive system healthy. Physical activity helps accelerate intestinal transit and can reduce the pressure inside the colon, thus helping to prevent the formation of diverticula.

Medication Management: Older adults often take multiple medications that can affect digestive health, such as opioids for pain management, which can cause constipation. Reviewing medications regularly with a healthcare provider can help minimize the impact of drugs on gut health.

Regular Medical Checkups: Since the symptoms of diverticulitis can be less pronounced in older individuals, regular checkups can help catch changes in gut health early. Diagnostic tests like colonoscopies can help monitor the health of the colon and detect diverticulosis before it progresses to diverticulitis.

Stress Management: Chronic stress can affect gut health and exacerbate many digestive problems, including diverticulitis. Mindfulness, meditation, and mild yoga are all techniques that help improve mental and physical health, especially in the elderly.

By adopting these lifestyle changes, older adults can not only reduce the risk of developing diverticulitis but also improve their overall gut health, enhancing their quality of life as they age. Awareness and proactive management are key in navigating the complexities of aging and maintaining a healthy digestive system.

Diverticulosis vs. Diverticulitis: Knowing the Difference

Understanding the distinction between diverticulosis and diverticulitis is crucial for managing gut health, especially as it pertains to symptom management and the prevention of flareups. Both conditions relate to the formation of small pouches, or diverticula, in the wall of the colon, but the similarity largely ends there, with each condition presenting different implications for health and requiring different management strategies.

Diverticulosis refers to the mere presence of diverticula in the colon. These pouches are typically benign and asymptomatic, and many people are unaware they have them. The formation of these pockets is generally attributed to a combination of age-related structural changes in the digestive tract, increased intestinal pressure from prolonged constipation, or a diet low in fiber. The walls of the intestines weaken over time, particularly under the strain of moving hard, low fiber stool, which contributes to the formation of these pouches. For most, diverticulosis is discovered incidentally during medical procedures or tests for other conditions, such as a colonoscopy.

In contrast, diverticulitis occurs when one or more of the diverticula become inflamed or infected. This transition from a harmless anatomical irregularity to a painful and potentially serious condition can be triggered by a small tear in the diverticulum, allowing bacteria from the intestine to infiltrate the walls. Diverticulitis symptoms include severe stomach discomfort, fever, nausea, and a noticeable shift in bowel patterns. This ailment can range in severity from minor episodes that can be treated with diet modifications and antibiotics to severe bouts that may necessitate hospitalization or surgery.

Understanding these two conditions and their interrelation is key to both treatment and prevention. For those diagnosed with diverticulosis, the goal is to prevent the progression of diverticulitis. This is primarily achieved through dietary management—increasing the intake of fiber to reduce the strain and pressure in the colon, thus lowering the risk of pouch inflammation or infection. Fiber rich fruits, vegetables, and whole grains soften and make feces easier to pass, reducing the pressure that causes diverticula in the first place.

For those who develop diverticulitis, treatment may involve antibiotics to clear up the infection, a temporary shift to a low fiber diet to allow the colon to heal, and, in more severe cases, surgical interventions may be necessary to resolve complications like perforations or abscesses.

Moreover, an understanding of these conditions not only aids in prevention but also in the early detection of symptoms that could indicate a worsening situation. Those with diverticulosis should be vigilant for signs of diverticulitis, as early treatment can prevent complications and lead to better outcomes. Early contact with a healthcare professional at the outset of symptoms, such as growing stomach discomfort, fever, or changes in bowel habits, can provide rapid and efficient therapies.

In educating individuals about these conditions, it's essential to emphasize the impact of dietary and lifestyle choices on their progression and management. Such knowledge empowers individuals to take control of their health, making informed decisions that can significantly affect their quality of life. It also reduces anxiety and fear by demystifying the conditions and providing clear guidance on how to live with or prevent them effectively.

Ultimately, the key takeaway is that while diverticulosis and diverticulitis are related, they represent different stages of a disease process that can largely be controlled through proactive health and dietary practices. By embracing a lifestyle that supports optimal digestive health, individuals can not only prevent the progression of diverticulosis to diverticulitis but also enhance their overall wellbeing.

Why Your Diet Matters More Than Ever

In the pursuit of maintaining optimal gut health and managing conditions such as diverticulitis, diet plays a pivotal role that cannot be overstated. The foods we consume directly influence the function and health of our gastrointestinal system, particularly as we age. A well- balanced diet high in particular nutrients can help avoid common digestive diseases and manage the symptoms of chronic illnesses such as diverticulitis.

The interactions between food and the microbiome—the large population of bacteria that live in our digestive tracts—are the basis of the relationship between diet and gut health. These microbes play critical roles in digestion, immune function, and inflammation regulation. An imbalance in these microbial populations can lead to dysbiosis, a disrupted microbial state that is often linked with numerous digestive disorders, including diverticulitis.

For individuals with diverticulosis, a diet high in fiber is particularly beneficial. Fiber raises the weight of the stool and shortens its transit time through the colon, lowering pressure inside the digestive system and lowering the risk of developing new diverticula or inflaming existing ones. Some foods high in soluble fiber that can help soften stool and lessen the need for straining include oats, peas, beans, apples, citrus fruits, carrots, barley, and psyllium. Insoluble fiber, which gives the stool weight and speeds up food passage through the stomach and intestines, is present in whole grains, wheat bran, nuts, beans, and vegetables like potatoes, cauliflower, and green beans.

Beyond fiber, a diet rich in fruits, vegetables, and whole grains provides antioxidants and anti-inflammatory compounds that can protect the gut lining and reduce the risk of inflammation. It is also advisable to reduce your intake of red meat and processed meals, which have been linked to an increased risk of diverticulitis and other digestive issues. These foods are often high in fat and sugar, which can exacerbate inflammation in the gut.

Hydration is another crucial aspect of a diet geared towards optimal gut health. Sufficient fluid intake ensures that the fiber consumed can perform its function effectively. Water allows the fiber to pass more easily through the digestive tract, lowering the probability of constipation and the tension that can contribute to diverticulitis flareups.

For those already managing diverticulitis, dietary recommendations may shift during periods of active inflammation. During a flareup, a low fiber diet may be advised to allow the colon to heal. Foods such as white rice, white bread, and meat provide little fiber and are easier on the colon. Once the inflammation subsides, a gradual reintroduction of fiber can help in preventing future episodes.

It is also worth noting the importance of avoiding certain foods that can irritate the gut or contribute to diverticulitis symptoms. Nuts, popcorn, and seeds were traditionally thought to pose risks; however, recent studies suggest they may not contribute to flareups as once believed. Nonetheless, individual tolerance can vary, and it is important for patients to monitor their own responses to these foods.

Adopting a Mediterranean diet, which is heavy in fruits, vegetables, whole grains, seafood, and healthy fats (such as olive oil) but low in red meat and processed foods, has been demonstrated to assist patients with diverticulitis. This diet not only enhances digestive health but also aids in weight maintenance and reduces the risk of chronic diseases.

Implementing dietary changes can be challenging, especially for those accustomed to different eating habits. It is frequently good to talk with a nutritionist or dietitian, who may give tailored advice based on specific health requirements and tastes. This professional assistance can ensure that dietary plans are nutritionally balanced and sustainable in the long term.

Common Dietary Missteps and How to Avoid Them

Navigating dietary choices can be particularly challenging for those prone to or managing diverticulitis, as certain foods can exacerbate symptoms and lead to painful flareups. Understanding the common dietary missteps that aggravate this condition is key to maintaining gut health and preventing discomfort. Here, we explore several dietary errors often made and offer practical strategies to avoid these pitfalls, ensuring a diet that supports rather than harms the gut.

One of the most frequent errors is the inadequate intake of fiber. Fiber is essential for bulking up the stool and fostering regular bowel movements, both of which serve to relieve colon pressure. However, a normal Western diet is generally lacking in fiber, which can cause constipation and, as a result, increased intestinal pressure. This pressure can cause diverticula to form and potentially become inflamed. To avoid this, individuals should aim to consume a balanced amount of both soluble and insoluble fiber. Foods that contain soluble fiber, which dissolves in water to produce a gel like material, include oats, lentils, apples, and berries. Insoluble fiber, which does not dissolve in water and helps add bulk to the stool, can be found in whole grains, nuts, and many vegetables. Gradually increasing fiber intake and consuming adequate water can prevent the bloating and gas sometimes associated with dietary fiber adjustments.

Another common misstep is consuming a diet high in red meat and processed foods, which are low in fiber and high in fats, which can trigger diverticulitis flareups. Studies have shown that these types of foods can not only trigger inflammation in the colon but also contribute to the development of further diverticula. Instead, incorporating lean proteins like poultry, fish, and plant Based sources can reduce these risks. Omega3 fatty acid rich fish, such as mackerel and salmon, are especially advantageous since they have anti Inflammatory qualities that enhance colon health.

Many people also make the mistake of eating large meals that overload the digestive system, particularly during flareups when the colon needs to heal. Eating more often and in smaller portions can assist in better managing these symptoms by reducing the amount of work the colon has to undertake at any given time. This approach allows the digestive system to process food more efficiently, minimizing the risk of constipation and the strain that exacerbates diverticulitis.

Consumption of specific types of lipids is another area where errors are common. Trans and saturated fats, which are commonly present in baked products, fried meals, and some margarine, can cause inflammation in the stomach. On the other hand, monounsaturated and polyunsaturated fats—found in olive oil, nuts, and avocados—can have an anti-inflammatory effect. Selecting the proper fats is crucial for preserving intestinal health and averting instances of diverticulitis.

Furthermore, reliance on laxatives for constipation relief can create dependency and worsen gut health over time. While occasional use may be necessary, it's better to rely on a high fiber diet and ample fluid intake to regulate bowel movements naturally. For those who struggle with regularity, speaking to a healthcare provider about gentler alternatives like stool softeners or bulk forming agents may be beneficial.

Alcohol and caffeine consumption is another common error among individuals prone to diverticulitis. Both substances can irritate the digestive tract and exacerbate symptoms. Moderation is key, and for those frequently experiencing flareups, it might be advisable to eliminate these substances entirely.

Lastly, ignoring food sensitivities and allergies can lead to repeated gut irritation, which can inflame diverticula and lead to severe complications. It is crucial for individuals to pay attention to how their bodies react to certain foods and to adjust their diets accordingly. This might involve cutting out gluten, lactose, or other irritants that trigger symptoms.

By understanding and avoiding these common dietary errors, individuals with diverticulitis can better manage their symptoms and reduce the likelihood of flareups. Incorporating a balanced, nutrient rich diet tailored to individual needs and sensitivities not only supports gut health but also enhances overall wellbeing.

Maintaining an open dialogue with healthcare providers about diet and symptom management can also provide crucial support, helping to finetune dietary strategies that work for each unique individual. Through careful dietary management, the challenges of living with diverticulitis can be significantly mitigated, allowing individuals to lead healthier and more comfortable lives.

Scan the QR Code and access your 3 bonuses in digital format

🔥 **Bonus 1: SUPPLEMENT GUIDE**

🔥 **Bonus 2: DAILY MENTAL HEALTH TIPS**

🔥 **Bonus 3: 90Day Meal Plan with Adjustments and Tips**

Scan the QR Code and access your 3 bonuses in digital format

2

HOW TO MANAGE FLARE UPS

Managing diverticulitis effectively hinges on the ability to recognize the early signs of a flare-up. Prompt detection and response can greatly mitigate the severity of the symptoms and may prevent the need for more intensive medical intervention. Individuals who are familiar with the symptoms associated with diverticulitis are better equipped to take swift action, ensuring that they manage their condition before it escalates.

A flare-up of diverticulitis typically begins with subtle changes that may be easy to overlook. One of the most common initial symptoms is an increase in cramping or pain in the lower left side of the abdomen. This pain may start off as mild and worsen over a period of hours or days. Unlike regular stomach aches or cramping, this pain persists and often intensifies with movement or when pressure is applied to the area. Individuals may find that certain activities, such as bending over or walking, exacerbate the discomfort, providing a key indicator that this is not a typical digestive upset.

Recognizing Early Warning Signs

Another early warning sign of a diverticulitis flare-up is a change in bowel habits. This could manifest as either new onset constipation or, less commonly, diarrhea. The development of constipation can be particularly concerning as it increases pressure in the colon, which can aggravate the inflamed diverticula. On the other hand, diarrhea may indicate that the body is attempting to clear out an infection or inflammation in the digestive tract. Monitoring these changes in bowel patterns can be critical in recognizing the early stages of a flare-up.

2

HOW TO MANAGE FLARE UPS

Managing diverticulitis effectively hinges on the ability to recognize the early signs of a flareup. Prompt detection and response can greatly mitigate the severity of the symptoms and may prevent the need for more intensive medical intervention. Individuals who are familiar with the symptoms associated with diverticulitis are better equipped to take swift action, ensuring that they manage their condition before it escalates.

A flareup of diverticulitis typically begins with subtle changes that may be easy to overlook. One of the most common initial symptoms is an increase in cramping or pain in the lower left side of the abdomen. This pain may start off as mild and worsen over a period of hours or days. Unlike regular stomach aches or cramping, this pain persists and often intensifies with movement or when pressure is applied to the area. Individuals may find that certain activities, such as bending over or walking, exacerbate the discomfort, providing a key indicator that this is not a typical digestive upset.

Recognizing Early Warning Signs

Another early warning sign of a diverticulitis flareup is a change in bowel habits. This could manifest as either new onset constipation or, less commonly, diarrhea. The development of constipation can be particularly concerning as it increases pressure in the colon, which can aggravate the inflamed diverticula. On the other hand, diarrhea may indicate that the body is attempting to clear out an infection or inflammation in the digestive tract. Monitoring these changes in bowel patterns can be critical in recognizing the early stages of a flareup.

Nausea and a general feeling of being unwell often accompany these changes in bowel habits and abdominal pain. Some individuals may experience a low-grade fever, signaling an inflammatory or infectious process within the body. This combination of symptoms—pain, altered bowel habits, nausea, and fever—should prompt immediate attention and possibly a consultation with a healthcare professional.

For those managing diverticulitis, being vigilant about these symptoms is key to early intervention. It is recommended that you maintain a symptom journal in which you record any changes in bowel habits, stomach discomfort, and other relevant symptoms, along with their frequency, severity, and duration. This record can be invaluable during doctor's visits, providing clear data points that can assist in the diagnosis and management of the condition.

Encouraging individuals to understand and monitor these symptoms empowers them to manage their health proactively. Recognizing the early signs of a diverticulitis flareup not only facilitates timely medical intervention but also encourages individuals to make immediate adjustments to their diet and lifestyle to mitigate symptoms. For example, at the first sign of increased abdominal pain or changes in bowel habits, reducing fiber intake temporarily can help minimize bowel movements and allow the colon to rest. Increasing fluid intake can also be beneficial, especially if constipation is present.

Moreover, individuals experiencing symptoms should evaluate their recent dietary choices. If a recent increase in the consumption of trigger foods—such as red meats, fried foods, or high fat items—coincides with the onset of symptoms, this could provide further evidence of a flareup. Understanding this correlation can help individuals make more informed dietary choices in the future.

To manage diverticulitis flareups, avoid using over the counter nonsteroidal anti-inflammatory medicines (NSAIDs) like ibuprofen or aspirin, which can increase gastrointestinal irritation and bleeding. Instead, individuals should consult with healthcare providers about safer pain management options that do not compromise gut health.

In addition to recognizing and responding to early symptoms, individuals with diverticulitis should maintain regular communication with their healthcare providers. This relationship ensures that they receive guidance tailored to their specific health needs, particularly during a flareup. Healthcare providers can offer advice on adjusting medications, managing diet during a flareup, and identifying when medical intervention may be necessary, such as antibiotics or, in severe cases, hospitalization.

Finally, being able to detect early indicators of a diverticulitis flareup and responding appropriately can have a substantial influence on the condition's outcome. Individuals with diverticulitis may actively manage their symptoms and retain a greater quality of life by remaining informed, keeping detailed records, and communicating openly with healthcare specialists.

Dietary Adjustments During Flare Ups

During a flareup of diverticulitis, making immediate dietary adjustments is crucial to alleviating symptoms and aiding recovery. The dietary approach during this sensitive time contrasts significantly with the usual high fiber diet recommended for maintaining gut health. Instead, a temporary switch to a low fiber or even liquid diet may be required to minimize the strain on the digestive system and allow the colon to recover.

When diverticulitis symptoms appear, such as acute abdominal discomfort, fever, and changes in bowel habits, the first approach is usually to follow a clear liquid diet. This initial phase helps rest the bowel. Consumables in this diet include broth, clear juices like apple or cranberry, ice pops, and gelatin desserts. These items ensure hydration and provide some energy without taxing the digestive system. This liquid diet is typically recommended for a few days or until symptoms begin to subside.

As symptoms improve, patients can gradually transition to a more substantial but still gentle diet, often referred to as a low fiber diet. Foods that are simple to digest and won't aggravate the inflamed diverticula fall under this category. Suitable foods for this stage include:

White bread, pasta, and rice: These refined carbohydrates are low in fiber and gentler on the gut compared to their wholegrain counterparts.

Cooked vegetables: Soft cooked carrots, green beans, spinach, and pumpkins are examples. It's crucial to avoid vegetables that might contain seeds or skin, as these can be difficult to digest.

Low fiber fruits: Bananas, cantaloupe, and honeydew melon are recommended. Like vegetables, fruits should be consumed without skins, and seedless varieties should be chosen.

Eggs and poultry: Scrambled eggs, chicken, or turkey, cooked without added fat and seasoned minimally, provide necessary proteins without adding fiber.

Potatoes: Well-cooked and without skins, potatoes are a good source of energy and are easy on the digestive tract.

During this transition period, it is important to avoid certain foods that could exacerbate symptoms or hinder the healing process. Foods to avoid include:

Raw fruits and vegetables: The fiber content, especially in unpeeled or uncooked forms, can be too harsh on a sensitive digestive system.

Whole grains: While generally healthy, whole grains like brown rice, quinoa, and whole wheat contain high levels of fiber, which could irritate the colon during a flareup.

Nuts and seeds: These can get trapped in the diverticula and cause irritation or further inflammation.

Dairy products: For some people, dairy products can exacerbate diarrhea and discomfort, especially if they are lactose intolerant.

Fatty, fried, and spicy foods: Such items can stimulate the intestines and worsen symptoms of pain and cramping.

It's also advisable to limit the consumption of caffeine and alcohol during this time, as they can stimulate the gut and may worsen symptoms like diarrhea and abdominal pain.

As the patient recovers and symptoms continue to diminish, they can gradually reintroduce more fiber into their diet. However, this reintroduction should be slow and monitored closely. The goal is to eventually return to a high fiber diet to help prevent future episodes of diverticulitis, but only once the inflammation has resolved sufficiently.

During this period, consulting with a healthcare physician or a dietitian can give individualized advice depending on the severity of the symptoms and your specific dietary requirements. This professional assistance may help guarantee that the diet not only relieves symptoms but also promotes general health and wellbeing throughout recovery.

Foods to Avoid

When managing diverticulitis, understanding which foods to avoid is just as crucial as knowing what to eat. Certain foods can exacerbate symptoms or trigger flareups by irritating the already sensitive lining of the colon or by becoming trapped in the diverticula, small pouches in the colon wall. Avoiding these foods during flareups and even during periods of remission can help maintain gut health and prevent further complications.

One major category of foods to avoid includes those that are high in certain types of fiber, particularly insoluble fiber, during a flareup. While a high fiber diet is generally recommended to prevent diverticulitis, foods with a high amount of insoluble fiber can aggravate symptoms when the condition is active. Insoluble fiber does not dissolve in water and adds bulk to the stool, which can be beneficial under normal circumstances, but during a diverticulitis flareup, it can cause painful pressure as it moves through the inflamed sections of the colon. Foods high in this type of fiber include whole grains such as bulgur and barley and fibrous vegetables such as broccoli, Brussels sprouts, and green peas.

Nuts and seeds have traditionally been flagged as problematic for individuals with diverticulitis because they are thought to get stuck in the diverticula. Although recent studies suggest that nuts and seeds might not be as harmful as once thought, many healthcare providers still recommend that patients avoid these foods during flareups until more definitive research is available. This includes all types of nuts, as well as seeds found in fruits vegetables, and those used as dietary supplements like flaxseed.

Corn, including popcorn, is another food to avoid. Like nuts and seeds, the small, hard kernels have the potential to become lodged in the diverticula. Corn is also high in insoluble fiber, which, as previously noted, can exacerbate symptoms during an active episode of diverticulitis by increasing bowel pressure and irritation.

Fruits with skins and seeds can also pose problems. These include berries such as raspberries and strawberries, which contain small seeds that can enter diverticula and cause irritation. Other problematic fruits include apples, pears, and figs, which have skins and seeds that are difficult to digest fully and might exacerbate symptoms.

In addition to fibrous foods, fatty and fried foods are particularly hard on the digestive system, especially during a diverticulitis flareup. High fat foods can stimulate contractions of the colon, potentially leading to increased abdominal pain and discomfort. This category includes fast foods, pastries, rich creams, and any food cooked in oil at high temperatures.

While spicy foods add taste to meals, they can also irritate the digestive tract and increase diverticulitis symptoms. Capsaicin, the heat producing component in chili peppers, can induce gastrointestinal pain and diarrhea in sensitive individuals, worsening the problem. Those suffering from diverticulitis are often advised to avoid spicy dishes until their system has healed and symptoms have subsided.

Red meat is harder to digest and can increase the inflammatory response in the body, which is not ideal when trying to manage diverticulitis. Digesting red meat also produces certain substances that may contribute to inflammation, further irritating the colon. During episodes of diverticulitis, it is best to limit red meat consumption and opt for easier to digest proteins like poultry or fish.

Lastly, dairy products can be problematic for some individuals, particularly those who are lactose intolerant. For these people, consuming dairy can lead to additional gas, bloating, and diarrhea, which can further irritate the colon during periods of inflammation. Even for those who are not lactose intolerant, dairy products can contribute to discomfort due to their high fat content, especially if consuming full fat versions.

Avoiding these specific foods can significantly impact the management of diverticulitis by reducing the risk of aggravating the colon during a flareup. It is also beneficial for long term management to moderate the intake of these foods even during periods of remission to maintain overall gut health. Making these dietary changes can help reduce the frequency and severity of diverticulitis symptoms, promoting a healthier, more comfortable life.

Gut Soothing Foods

In the management of diverticulitis, particularly during and following flareups, selecting foods that soothe the gut is as important as avoiding those that aggravate it. Certain foods are known for their gentle effects on the digestive system, promoting healing and reducing inflammation. Incorporating these gut soothing foods into one's diet can aid significantly in the recovery process and help maintain long term digestive health.

During the initial recovery phase of a diverticulitis flareup, when the gut is most tender, the focus should be on foods that are easy to digest and low in fiber. As the inflammation subsides, these foods can help restore normal digestive function without overtaxing the digestive system.

Cooked fruits and vegetables are excellent choices during this period. Cooking breaks down the fibers in these foods, making them easier for a sensitive gut to handle. For example, carrots, squash, pumpkins, and potatoes can be boiled or steamed until they are soft and free of any tough skins or seeds. Apples and pears can be baked or turned into applesauce, which eliminates their fibrous skins and seeds, making them gentle on the gut.

Another category of gut soothing foods includes clear broths and soups. These are particularly beneficial immediately following a flareup. Broths provide hydration and essential nutrients without solid particles that could irritate the gut. Chicken or vegetable broth, strained to remove any solids, can serve as a soothing meal that provides some protein and minerals, aiding in recovery without stressing the digestive system.

Oatmeal is another excellent food for those recovering from diverticulitis. It's not only easy to digest but also contains soluble fiber, which helps to form a gel like substance in the gut, softening stools and improving bowel movement ease. Oatmeal can be made with water or nondairy milk to keep it light and easy on the stomach, and it should be cooked until very soft.

Yogurt, particularly types that contain live probiotics is beneficial for gut health. Probiotics are living bacteria that help restore the gut's natural equilibrium, which can be disturbed during diverticulitis. Eating yogurt can bring healthy bacteria into the digestive tract, which aids digestion and reduces inflammation. Lactose intolerant people should avoid lactose containing meals and take probiotic supplements instead.

Lean proteins such as chicken, turkey, and fish are crucial during the recovery phase as they provide the necessary nutrients without the fat content that can exacerbate symptoms. These proteins should be cooked simply—boiled, baked, or grilled without added fats or oils. The simplicity in preparation helps ensure these foods are digestible while still supporting bodily repair and maintenance.

When ingested in moderation, smooth nut butters like peanut or almond butter may be relaxing and contain protein and good fats. It is important to choose varieties that are smooth and free of any chunks or additives that could irritate the gut. These can be spread thinly on soft, white toast or added to oatmeal or yogurt for a nutrient boost.

Eggs are another versatile and gut friendly food, easy to digest and packed with protein, which can be crucial in healing. They can be prepared soft boiled, poached, or scrambled without milk or butter to keep them light and easy on the stomach.

Lastly, hydration plays a pivotal role in recovery from any digestive issue, including diverticulitis. Water is essential, but other fluids like herbal teas can be soothing as well. Peppermint and ginger tea, for example, contain natural anti-inflammatory effects that can help relax the digestive tract and relieve discomfort. These teas can reduce bloating and calm spasms in the gut, providing relief during recovery.

Incorporating these foods into the diet during and after a diverticulitis flareup can help soothe the gut, ease symptoms, and speed up the recovery process. As the gut heals, gradually reintroducing more fibrous foods is important, but this initial gentle approach can provide the foundation for stronger digestive health. It's also advisable to work with a healthcare provider or dietitian to tailor dietary choices to individual health needs and to adjust the diet as recovery progresses and gut health improves. This personalized approach ensures that the diet supports recovery and long-term health, helping prevent future digestive issues.

Hydration Tactics

Hydration is essential for managing diverticulitis and maintaining overall digestive health. Water is fundamental to various bodily functions, including digestion, as it helps to soften stools and facilitates smooth passage through the colon. This is particularly important in the prevention and management of diverticulitis, where ensuring easy bowel movements can help reduce pressure in the colon and minimize the risk of the diverticula becoming inflamed or infected.

For individuals with diverticulitis, maintaining adequate hydration is essential, especially during flareups when the risk of dehydration increases due to reduced fluid intake and, in some cases, increased fluid loss through diarrhea. Dehydration can exacerbate constipation, which in turn increases the chances of a diverticulitis attack by adding stress to the colon. Thus, ensuring a consistent and adequate intake of fluids is vital in managing the symptoms and preventing the progression of diverticulitis.

Water is the most effective source of hydration. It is advised that people drink at least eight 8ounce glasses of water every day, while this might vary depending on body size, activity level, and overall health. It's important to note that fluid needs increase when fiber intake is high, as fiber pulls water into the colon to form softer, bulkier stools. Therefore, those who are increasing their fiber intake to manage or prevent diverticulitis should also increase their water consumption.

Aside from water, other fluids can contribute to overall hydration. Herbal teas, such as chamomile or peppermint, are ideal alternatives since they may soothe the digestive tract. These teas provide a calming, anti-inflammatory benefit, which can be particularly helpful during flareups of diverticulitis. However, it is crucial to avoid teas that contain caffeine, as caffeine can stimulate the intestines, potentially worsening symptoms.

In certain situations, patients may struggle to consume enough water, particularly if they are not used to drinking a lot of water. One strategy to increase fluid intake is to incorporate foods with high water content into the diet. Foods such as cucumbers, tomatoes, strawberries, watermelon, and peaches contain significant amounts of water and can contribute to overall fluid intake. These foods also provide the added benefit of being rich in vitamins and minerals, supporting overall health.

Establishing a habit is also an efficient strategy to guarantee enough hydration. Drinking a glass of water when you wake up, before each meal, and in between meals can assist in spreading fluid intake throughout the day, making it easier to digest and absorb. Carrying a water bottle and sipping it throughout the day is another practical strategy to increase your water consumption. Setting phone reminders or utilizing water tracking apps might help people maintain good hydration habits.

It is also important for those managing diverticulitis to adjust their fluid intake based on their activity level and the climate. During hot weather or physical exercise, the body loses water through perspiration, which must be replaced by consuming more fluids. Failure to do so might result in dehydration, which can either cause or worsen diverticulitis symptoms.

While increasing fluid intake, it is essential to moderate the consumption of beverages that can be dehydrating or irritating to the gut. These include alcohol, sugary drinks, and caffeinated beverages. Alcohol can contribute to dehydration and also cause inflammation in the gut, which can worsen diverticulitis symptoms. Similarly, sugary drinks can lead to spikes in blood sugar and may contribute to obesity, which is a risk factor for diverticulitis. Caffeinated beverages, while mildly diuretic, can also irritate the digestive system.

For individuals recovering from a diverticulitis flareup, gradually reintroducing fluids other than water can be part of the recovery process. Starting with clear liquids like broth and then moving to more substantial fluids like fruit juices (without pulp) can help restore normal digestion and provide nutrients that may have been lacking during the flareup.

Medical Interventions

Diverticulitis is a condition characterized by the inflammation or infection of small pouches called diverticula that can form in the lining of the digestive system. The severity of diverticulitis can vary significantly, requiring different levels of medical intervention, from dietary management to urgent surgical procedures. Understanding when and how to seek medical intervention, manage the condition with appropriate medications, and handle emergency situations are critical aspects of dealing with this digestive disorder.

Medical interventions for diverticulitis depend largely on the severity and frequency of the episodes. Initially, for mild diverticulitis, treatment might involve dietary modifications such as a liquid diet to rest the bowel, along with a course of antibiotics to treat the infection. Patients are usually advised to monitor their condition closely and maintain communication with their healthcare provider.

For recurrent or severe cases, more intensive medical intervention may be necessary. This can include a longer duration of antibiotics, a more strictly monitored diet, or even hospitalization to manage pain and prevent further complications. If nonsurgical treatments fail or if complications arise, surgical interventions such as a partial colectomy might be recommended. This procedure involves the removal of the affected part of the colon, potentially preventing future episodes of diverticulitis.

When to See a doctor

It is crucial to consult a healthcare provider if you suspect diverticulitis or if you have been diagnosed with diverticulosis and begin to notice symptoms like abdominal pain, changes in bowel habits, or other related symptoms. Regular checkups can help manage the condition before it worsens.

Immediate medical attention should be sought if symptoms intensify or if you experience severe abdominal pain, high fever, or significant changes in bowel habits. These signs could indicate the progression of the disease or the onset of complications, which require prompt intervention to prevent more serious outcomes.

Medications and Treatments

The first line of treatment for uncomplicated diverticulitis often involves antibiotics to clear up the infection and nonopioid pain relievers to avoid exacerbating symptoms with medications that could cause constipation or additional gut irritation. Commonly prescribed antibiotics include ciprofloxacin in combination with metronidazole or amoxicillin clavulanate.

Alongside medication, a temporary shift to a clear liquid diet is usually recommended to allow the colon to heal. After symptoms improve, a gradual reintroduction of fiber helps restore normal bowel function and reduces the risk of future flareups.

For chronic or complicated cases, other medications, such as probiotics or anti-inflammatory drugs, might be used to manage symptoms and maintain gut health. Ongoing treatment strategies are often adjusted based on individual responses and the frequency of episodes.

Navigating Emergency Situations

Diverticulitis can sometimes lead to serious complications such as perforations in the colon, abscesses, or generalized infection (sepsis). These conditions require immediate emergency care. Symptoms that should prompt an urgent visit to the emergency room include:

- Sudden, severe abdominal pain
- High fever accompanied by chills
- Uncontrolled vomiting
- Evidence of an infection, such as pus or blood in the stool
-

Signs of shock such as fainting, rapid heart rate, or severe lightheadedness

In these scenarios, treatment may involve intravenous antibiotics, emergency surgery to remove the affected part of the colon, or drainage of abscesses if present. Timely medical response in such situations can be lifesaving and prevent long term complications.

3

RECIPES

Breakfast (25 Recipes)

Banana Oatmeal Smoothie

Ingredients:

- 1 ripe banana
- 1/2 cup rolled oats
- 1 cup milk (dairy or nondairy)
- 1 tablespoon honey or maple syrup
- 1/2 teaspoon cinnamon
- 1/2 teaspoon vanilla extract
- 1/4 cup Greek yogurt (optional for extra creaminess)

Instructions:

1. Combine all ingredients in a blender.
2. Blend until smooth and creamy.
3. Pour into a glass and serve immediately.

Nutritional Values (per serving):

- Calories: 300
- Fat: 5g
- Carbohydrates: 60g
- Protein: 10g

Egg White Scramble with Spinach

Ingredients:

- 4 egg whites
- 1 cup fresh spinach, chopped
- 1/4 cup chopped onion
- 1 tablespoon olive oil
- Salt and pepper to taste

Instructions:

1. Heat the olive oil in a nonstick skillet over medium heat.
2. Add the chopped onion and cook until translucent.
3. Add the spinach and cook until wilted.
4. Pour in the egg whites and scramble until cooked through.
5. Season with salt and pepper to taste.
6. Serve hot.

Nutritional Values (per serving):

- Calories: 120
- Fat: 7g
- Carbohydrates: 3g
- Protein: 12g

Ginger Pear Breakfast Salad

Ingredients:

- 2 ripe pears, sliced
- 1/2 teaspoon fresh ginger, grated
- 1/4 cup plain Greek yogurt
- 1 tablespoon honey
- 1 tablespoon lemon juice
- 1/4 cup granola (optional for added crunch)

Instructions:

1. In a small bowl, mix the Greek yogurt, honey, lemon juice, and grated ginger.
2. Arrange the pear slices on a plate.
3. Drizzle the yogurt mixture over the pears.
4. Top with granola if using.
5. Serve immediately.

Nutritional Values (per serving):

- Calories: 200
- Fat: 2g
- Carbohydrates: 45g
- Protein: 5g

Pumpkin Porridge

Ingredients:

- 1/2 cup rolled oats
- 1 cup milk (dairy or nondairy)
- 1/4 cup canned pumpkin puree
- 1 tablespoon honey or maple syrup
- 1/2 teaspoon cinnamon
- 1/4 teaspoon nutmeg

Instructions:

1. In a saucepan, combine the oats, milk, pumpkin puree, honey, cinnamon, and nutmeg.
2. Bring to a boil, then reduce heat and simmer for 57 minutes, stirring occasionally, until the oats are tender and the porridge is thick.
3. Serve hot, optionally topped with a sprinkle of cinnamon or a dollop of yogurt.

Nutritional Values (per serving):

- Calories: 220
- Fat: 4g
- Carbohydrates: 40g
- Protein: 6g

Soothing Rice Pudding

Ingredients:

- 1/2 cup white rice
- 4 cups milk (dairy or nondairy)
- 1/4 cup sugar
- 1 teaspoon vanilla extract
- 1/2 teaspoon ground cinnamon

Instructions:

1. In a large saucepan, combine the rice, milk, and sugar.
2. Bring to a boil over medium high heat, then reduce the heat to low and simmer, stirring frequently, for 3040 minutes, or until the rice is tender and the pudding is thickened.
3. Stir in the vanilla extract and ground cinnamon.
4. Serve warm or chilled.

Nutritional Values (per serving):

- Calories: 200
- Fat: 5g
- Carbohydrates: 35g
- Protein: 6g

Avocado and Egg Toast on Sourdough

Ingredients:

- 2 slices sourdough bread
- 1 ripe avocado
- 2 eggs
- 1 tablespoon olive oil
- Salt and pepper to taste

Instructions:

1. Toast the sourdough bread slices.
2. In a small bowl, mash the avocado with a fork and season with salt and pepper.
3. Heat the olive oil in a nonstick skillet over medium heat. Fry the eggs until the whites are set and the yolks are cooked to your liking.
4. Spread the mashed avocado on the toasted sourdough slices.
5. Top each slice with a fried egg.
6. Serve immediately.

Nutritional Values (per serving):

- Calories: 350
- Fat: 25g
- Carbohydrates: 28g
- Protein: 10g

Plain Greek Yogurt with Honey

Ingredients:

- 1 cup plain Greek yogurt
- 1 tablespoon honey
- Optional: fresh fruit or granola for topping

Instructions:

1. Place the Greek yogurt in a bowl.
2. Drizzle the honey over the yogurt.
3. Add optional toppings like fresh fruit or granola if desired.
4. Serve immediately.

Nutritional Values (per serving):

- Calories: 150
- Fat: 5g
- Carbohydrates: 18g
- Protein: 10g

Smooth Cottage Cheese with Blueberries

Ingredients:

- 1 cup cottage cheese
- 1/2 cup fresh or frozen blueberries
- 1 tablespoon honey or maple syrup (optional)

Instructions:

1. In a bowl, combine the cottage cheese and blueberries.
2. Drizzle with honey or maple syrup if desired.

Serve immediately.

Nutritional Values (per serving):

- Calories: 160
- Fat: 5g
- Carbohydrates: 15g
- Protein: 14g

Almond Butter and Banana on Toast

Ingredients:

- 2 slices whole grain bread
- 2 tablespoons almond butter
- 1 banana, sliced
- Optional: a sprinkle of cinnamon or chia seeds

Instructions:

1. Toast the slices of whole grain bread.
2. Spread almond butter evenly on each slice of toast.
3. Top with banana slices.
4. Sprinkle with cinnamon or chia seeds if desired.
5. Serve immediately.

Nutritional Values (per serving):

- Calories: 300
- Fat: 15g
- Carbohydrates: 35g
- Protein: 8g

Steamed Vegetable Omelette

Ingredients:

- 3 eggs
- 1/2 cup steamed mixed vegetables (such as bell peppers, spinach, and mushrooms)
- 1/4 cup shredded cheese (optional)
- 1 tablespoon olive oil

- Salt and pepper to taste

Instructions:

1. In a bowl, whisk the eggs with salt and pepper.
2. Heat the olive oil in a nonstick skillet over medium heat.
3. Pour the eggs into the skillet and cook until they begin to set.
4. Add the steamed vegetables and cheese (if using) on one half of the omelette.
5. Fold the other half of the omelette over the filling and cook until the eggs are fully set.
6. Serve hot.

Nutritional Values (per serving):

- Calories: 250
- Fat: 18g
- Carbohydrates: 5g
- Protein: 18g

Low-FODMAP Muesli

Ingredients:

- 1 cup rolled oats (gluten-free if needed)
- 1/4 cup shredded coconut (unsweetened)
- 1/4 cup sunflower seeds
- 1/4 cup pumpkin seeds

- 1/4 cup chopped walnuts
- 1/4 cup dried cranberries (no added sugar)
- 1 teaspoon cinnamon

Instructions:

1. In a large bowl, combine all ingredients and mix well.
2. Store in an airtight container.
3. Serve with lactose-free milk or yogurt and fresh berries.

Nutritional Values (per serving):

- Calories: 250
- Fat: 15g
- Carbohydrates: 25g
- Protein: 6g

Oatmeal Pancakes

Ingredients:

- 1 cup rolled oats
- 1 cup milk (dairy or non-dairy)
- 1 egg
- 1 tablespoon honey
- 1 teaspoon vanilla extract
- 1 teaspoon baking powder
- 1/2 teaspoon cinnamon
- Pinch of salt

Instructions:

1. In a blender, combine all ingredients and blend until smooth.
2. Heat a non-stick skillet over medium heat and lightly grease with oil.
3. Pour batter onto the skillet, forming small pancakes.
4. Cook until bubbles form on the surface, then flip and cook until golden brown.
5. Serve with fresh fruit and a drizzle of honey.

Nutritional Values (per serving):

- Calories: 200
- Fat: 5g
- Carbohydrates: 30g
- Protein: 8g

Homemade Granola with Rice Milk

Ingredients:

- 2 cups rolled oats
- 1/2 cup chopped almonds
- 1/2 cup shredded coconut
- 1/4 cup pumpkin seeds
- 1/4 cup sunflower seeds
- 2 tablespoons coconut oil, melted
- 2 tablespoons honey or maple syrup
- 1 teaspoon vanilla extract
- 1/2 cup dried cranberries
- Rice milk, for serving

Instructions:

1. Preheat your oven to 300°F (150°C) and line a baking sheet with parchment paper.
2. In a large bowl, combine the oats, almonds, shredded coconut, pumpkin seeds, and sunflower seeds.
3. In a separate bowl, mix the melted coconut oil, honey (or maple syrup), and vanilla extract.
4. Pour the wet ingredients over the dry ingredients and mix well.
5. Spread the granola mixture evenly on the prepared baking sheet.
6. Bake in the preheated oven for 2025 minutes, stirring occasionally, until golden and crisp.
7. Remove from the oven and stir in the dried cranberries.
8. Let the granola cool completely before serving with rice milk.

Nutritional Values (per serving, about 1/2 cup):

- Calories: 300

- Fat: 15g
- Carbohydrates: 34g
- Protein: 6g

Baked Sweet Potato with Yogurt

Ingredients:

- 1 large sweet potato
- 1/2 cup plain Greek yogurt (low fat or full fat based on preference)
- Optional toppings: a sprinkle of cinnamon, a drizzle of honey, or chopped nuts for added texture

Instructions:

1. Preheat your oven to 400°F (200°C).
2. Thoroughly wash the sweet potato and pierce it several times with a fork to allow steam to escape during cooking.
3. Place the sweet potato on a baking sheet lined with aluminum foil or parchment paper.
4. Bake in the preheated oven for 4550 minutes, or until the sweet potato is tender when pierced with a fork.
5. Remove the sweet potato from the oven and let it cool slightly.
6. Split the sweet potato open and fluff the inside with a fork.
7. Top the sweet potato with Greek yogurt. For additional flavor, sprinkle cinnamon, drizzle honey, or add chopped nuts.

Nutritional Values (per serving):

- Calories: 200
- Fat: 0.5g
- Carbohydrates: 45g
- Protein: 6g

Low - Fiber Bran Muffins

Ingredients:

- 1 cup wheat bran
- 1 cup low fiber all -purpose flour
- 1/2 cup sugar
- 1 teaspoon baking soda
- 1 teaspoon baking powder
- 1/2 teaspoon salt
- 1 cup buttermilk (or a nondairy milk with 1 tablespoon of vinegar to sour it)

- 1/3 cup vegetable oil
- 1 large egg

Instructions:

1. Preheat your oven to 375°F (190°C) and line a muffin tin with paper liners or lightly grease the cups.
2. In a large mixing bowl, combine the wheat bran, low fiber all -purpose flour, sugar, baking soda, baking powder, and salt.
3. In another bowl, whisk together the buttermilk, vegetable oil, and egg.
4. Add the wet ingredients to the dry ingredients and stir just until combined; the batter should still be slightly lumpy.
5. Spoon the batter into the prepared muffin tin, filling each cup about 2/3 full.
6. Bake in the preheated oven for 1520 minutes, or until a toothpick inserted into the center of a muffin comes out clean.
7. Remove the muffins from the oven and let them cool in the pan for 5 minutes before transferring them to a wire rack to cool completely.

Nutritional Values (per muffin):

- Calories: 180
- Fat: 8g
- Carbohydrates: 24g
- Protein: 4g

Tofu Scramble

Ingredients:

- 1 block (14 ounces) firm tofu, drained and crumbled
- 1 tablespoon olive oil
- 1/2 teaspoon turmeric
- 1 small onion, finely chopped
- 1/2 bell pepper, diced
- 1/2 teaspoon garlic powder
- Salt and pepper to taste
- Optional: chopped spinach, mushrooms, or tomatoes

Instructions:

1. Heat the olive oil in a nonstick skillet over medium heat.
2. Add the chopped onion and bell pepper. Sauté for about 5 minutes, or until the vegetables are soft.
3. Crumble the tofu into the skillet with your hands. Add the turmeric, garlic powder, salt, and pepper. Stir to combine.
4. Cook for 57 minutes, stirring frequently until the tofu is heated through and starts to get a slightly golden color.

5. If using optional vegetables, add them towards the end of cooking.
6. Serve hot, garnished with fresh herbs or a sprinkle of nutritional yeast.

Nutritional Values (per serving):

- Calories: 150
- Fat: 10g
- Carbohydrates: 6g
- Protein: 12g

Apple Cinnamon Porridge

Ingredients:

- 1 cup rolled oats
- 2 cups water or milk (dairy or nondairy)
- 1 medium apple, peeled and grated
- 1/2 teaspoon cinnamon
- 1 tablespoon honey or maple syrup (optional)
- A pinch of salt

Instructions:

1. In a medium saucepan, bring the water or milk to a boil.

2. Add the rolled oats and a pinch of salt. Reduce the heat to a simmer.
3. Stir in the grated apple and cinnamon. Cook, stirring occasionally, for about 57 minutes, or until the oats are soft and the porridge has thickened.
4. Remove from heat and stir in honey or maple syrup if using.
5. Serve warm, with an extra sprinkle of cinnamon on top if desired.

Nutritional Values (per serving):

- Calories: 220
- Fat: 3g
- Carbohydrates: 40g
- Protein: 6g

Egg Custard

Ingredients:

- 2 cups milk (dairy or nondairy)
- 4 large eggs
- 1/3 cup granulated sugar
- 1 teaspoon vanilla extract
- A pinch of salt
- Nutmeg for sprinkling on top (optional)

Instructions:

1. Preheat your oven to 325°F (165°C).
2. In a saucepan, heat the milk just until it starts to bubble around the edges. Remove from heat.
3. In a large bowl, whisk together the eggs, sugar, vanilla extract, and salt until well combined.
4. Gradually add the heated milk to the egg mixture, stirring continuously to avoid cooking the eggs.
5. Strain the mixture through a fine sieve into a large measuring cup or a bowl with a pour spout to ensure a smooth custard.
6. Pour the mixture into individual ramekins or a larger baking dish.
7. Place the ramekins or baking dish in a larger baking pan and carefully pour hot water into the pan to come halfway up the sides of the ramekins or dish.
8. Sprinkle the top of each custard with a pinch of nutmeg if desired.
9. Bake in the preheated oven for 4550 minutes, or until the custard is set but still slightly jiggly in the center.
10. Remove from the water bath and let cool. Serve chilled or at room temperature.

Nutritional Values (per serving):

- Calories: 180
- Fat: 9g
- Carbohydrates: 18g
- Protein: 8g

Polenta with Honey

Ingredients:

- 1 cup polenta (coarse cornmeal)
- 4 cups water or milk (dairy or nondairy)
- 1/4 teaspoon salt
- 2 tablespoons honey
- 1 tablespoon butter or a dairy free alternative

Instructions:

1. In a large saucepan, bring the water or milk to a boil. Add the salt.
2. Gradually whisk in the polenta to prevent lumps.
3. Reduce the heat to low and simmer, stirring frequently, for about 2025 minutes, or until the polenta is thick and creamy.
4. Stir in the honey and butter until well combined.
5. Serve warm, optionally topped with a drizzle of honey.

Nutritional Values (per serving):

- Calories: 200
- Fat: 4g
- Carbohydrates: 40g
- Protein: 4g

Quinoa Breakfast Bowl

Ingredients:

- 1 cup quinoa, rinsed
- 2 cups water or milk (dairy or nondairy)
- 1/2 teaspoon cinnamon
- 1 apple, diced
- 1/4 cup raisins
- 1/4 cup chopped nuts (such as walnuts or almonds, optional)
- 1 tablespoon honey or maple syrup
- Fresh berries or banana slices for topping

Instructions:

1. In a medium saucepan, bring the water or milk to a boil. Add the rinsed quinoa and cinnamon, then reduce the heat to a simmer.
2. Cover and cook for 1520 minutes, or until the quinoa is tender and the liquid has been absorbed.
3. Remove from heat and let it sit covered for 5 minutes. Fluff with a fork.
4. Stir in the diced apple, raisins, and chopped nuts if using. Drizzle with honey or maple syrup to sweeten.
5. Serve warm, topped with fresh berries or banana slices for added sweetness and a boost of vitamins.

Nutritional Values (per serving):

- Calories: 320
- Fat: 5g
- Carbohydrates: 60g
- Protein: 8g

Coconut Rice with Mango

Ingredients:

- 1 cup jasmine or basmati rice, rinsed
- 1 cup coconut milk
- 1 cup water
- 1/2 teaspoon salt
- 1 ripe mango, peeled and diced
- Fresh lime zest and juice to taste
- Chopped fresh cilantro or mint for garnish

Instructions:

1. In a saucepan, combine the rinsed rice, coconut milk, water, and salt. Bring the mixture to a boil.
2. Reduce the heat to low, cover, and simmer for 1820 minutes, or until the rice is tender and the liquid is absorbed.
3. Remove from heat and let it stand covered for 10 minutes.
4. Fluff the rice with a fork and gently stir in the diced mango, lime zest, and lime juice.
5. Serve the coconut rice warm or at room temperature, garnished with chopped cilantro or mint for a fresh flavor contrast.

Nutritional Values (per serving):

- Calories: 270
- Fat: 8g
- Carbohydrates: 45g
- Protein: 4g

Rice Cakes with Avocado Spread

Ingredients:

- 4 rice cakes (plain or lightly salted)
- 1 ripe avocado
- 1 tablespoon lemon juice
- 1/2 teaspoon salt
- 1/4 teaspoon black pepper
- Optional toppings: cherry tomatoes, radish slices, microgreens, or a sprinkle of sesame seeds

Instructions:

1. In a small bowl, mash the avocado with a fork until smooth.
2. Add the lemon juice, salt, and black pepper to the mashed avocado and mix well to combine.
3. Spread the avocado mixture evenly over the rice cakes.
4. Add optional toppings like cherry tomatoes, radish slices, microgreens, or sesame seeds for extra flavor and nutrition.
5. Serve immediately to enjoy the crisp texture of the rice cakes paired with the creamy avocado spread.

Nutritional Values (per serving of 2 rice cakes with avocado spread):

- Calories: 220
- Fat: 14g
- Carbohydrates: 22g
- Protein: 3g

Sweet Corn Porridge

Ingredients:

- 1 cup fresh or frozen sweet corn kernels
- 1 cup water
- 1 cup milk (dairy or nondairy)
- 1/2 teaspoon salt
- 1 tablespoon honey or maple syrup (optional)
- Ground cinnamon or nutmeg for garnish (optional)

Instructions:

1. In a medium saucepan, combine the sweet corn kernels, water, milk, and salt. Bring to a boil over medium heat.
2. Reduce the heat and simmer for 1015 minutes, stirring occasionally, until the corn is tender and the mixture thickens to a porridgelike consistency.
3. Remove from heat and stir in honey or maple syrup if using, for added sweetness.
4. Serve warm, garnished with a sprinkle of ground cinnamon or nutmeg if desired, for an extra flavor boost.

Nutritional Values (per serving):

- Calories: 180
- Fat: 5g
- Carbohydrates: 30g
- Protein: 6gHerbed Ricotta on Gluten free Toast

Herbed Ricotta on Gluten-free Toast

Ingredients:

- 4 slices gluten free bread
- 1 cup ricotta cheese
- 2 tablespoons fresh basil, chopped
- 2 tablespoons fresh parsley, chopped
- 1 tablespoon fresh chives, chopped
- 1 tablespoon olive oil
- Salt and pepper to taste
- Optional: cherry tomatoes or avocado slices for topping

Instructions:

1. Toast the gluten free bread slices until golden brown.
2. In a bowl, mix the ricotta cheese with the chopped basil, parsley, chives, olive oil, salt, and pepper until well combined.

3. Spread the herbed ricotta mixture evenly over the toasted bread slices.
4. Top with cherry tomatoes or avocado slices if desired for extra flavor and nutrition.
5. Serve immediately.

Nutritional Values (per serving):

- Calories: 200
- Fat: 10g
- Carbohydrates: 20g
- Protein: 8

Low - FODMAP Smoothie Bowl

Ingredients:

- 1/2 cup lactose free yogurt or coconut yogurt
- 1/2 banana (low FODMAP portion)
- 1/2 cup frozen strawberries
- 1/4 cup almond milk or lactose free milk
- 1 tablespoon chia seeds
- 1/4 cup gluten free granola
- Fresh berries and sliced kiwi for topping (optional)

Instructions:

1. In a blender, combine the lactose free yogurt or coconut yogurt, banana, frozen strawberries, almond milk, and chia seeds. Blend until smooth.
2. Pour the smoothie into a bowl.
3. Top with gluten free granola and fresh berries or sliced kiwi if desired.
4. Serve immediately with a spoon.

Nutritional Values (per serving):

- Calories: 300
- Fat: 10g
- Carbohydrates: 45g
- Protein: 8g

Lunch (25 Recipes)

Roasted Butternut Squash Soup

Ingredients:

- 1 large butternut squash, peeled, seeded, and cubed
- 2 tablespoons olive oil

- 1 large onion, chopped
- 3 cloves garlic, minced
- 4 cups vegetable broth
- 1 teaspoon ground cumin
- 1/2 teaspoon ground nutmeg
- Salt and pepper to taste
- Fresh parsley for garnish

Instructions:

1. Preheat your oven to 400°F (200°C).
2. Toss the butternut squash cubes with 1 tablespoon of olive oil, salt, and pepper. Spread evenly on a baking sheet.
3. Roast in the preheated oven for 2530 minutes, or until the squash is tender and caramelized.
4. In a large pot, heat the remaining olive oil over medium heat. Add the onion and garlic, and sauté until soft and fragrant.
5. Add the roasted squash, vegetable broth, cumin, and nutmeg. Bring to a boil, then reduce heat and simmer for 1520 minutes.
6. Use an immersion blender to puree the soup until smooth. Adjust seasoning with salt and pepper.
7. Serve hot, garnished with fresh parsley.

Nutritional Values (per serving):

- Calories: 180
- Fat: 7g
- Carbohydrates: 30g
- Protein: 3g

Turmeric Chicken Soup

Ingredients:

- 2 chicken breasts, cooked and shredded
- 1 large onion, chopped
- 2 carrots, diced
- 2 celery stalks, diced
- 3 cloves garlic, minced
- 1 tablespoon fresh ginger, grated
- 1 teaspoon ground turmeric
- 6 cups chicken broth
- 1 tablespoon olive oil
- Salt and pepper to taste
- Fresh cilantro for garnish

Instructions:

1. In a large pot, heat the olive oil over medium heat. Add the onion, carrots, celery, garlic, and ginger. Sauté until the vegetables are tender.
2. Stir in the turmeric and cook for another minute.

3. Add the chicken broth and bring to a boil.
4. Reduce heat and simmer for 20 minutes.
5. Add the shredded chicken and cook until heated through.
6. Season with salt and pepper.
7. Serve hot, garnished with fresh cilantro.

Nutritional Values (per serving):

- Calories: 200
- Fat: 5g
- Carbohydrates: 15g
- Protein: 25g

Grilled Cheese on Gluten - Free Bread

Ingredients:

- 4 slices gluten free bread
- 4 slices cheddar cheese
- 2 tablespoons butter

Instructions:

1. Heat a skillet over medium heat.
2. Butter one side of each bread slice.

3. Place two slices of bread, buttered side down, in the skillet.
4. Top each slice with two slices of cheese.
5. Place the remaining bread slices on top, buttered side up.
6. Cook until the bread is golden brown and the cheese is melted, flipping once.
7. Serve hot.

Nutritional Values (per serving):

- Calories: 350
- Fat: 25g
- Carbohydrates: 25g
- Protein: 10g

Simple Quinoa Salad

Ingredients:

- 1 cup quinoa, rinsed
- 2 cups water
- 1 cup cherry tomatoes, halved
- 1 cucumber, diced
- 1/4 cup red onion, finely chopped
- 1/4 cup fresh parsley, chopped
- 1/4 cup feta cheese, crumbled (optional)
- 3 tablespoons olive oil

- 2 tablespoons lemon juice
- Salt and pepper to taste

Instructions:

1. In a medium saucepan, bring the water to a boil. Add the quinoa, reduce heat, and simmer for 1520 minutes, or until the water is absorbed and the quinoa is tender.
2. Fluff the quinoa with a fork and let it cool to room temperature.
3. In a large bowl, combine the cooled quinoa, cherry tomatoes, cucumber, red onion, parsley, and feta cheese.
4. In a small bowl, whisk together the olive oil, lemon juice, salt, and pepper. Pour over the salad and toss to combine.
5. Serve chilled or at room temperature.

Nutritional Values (per serving):

- Calories: 250
- Fat: 14g
- Carbohydrates: 24g
- Protein: 7g

Tuna Salad Stuffed Avocado

Ingredients:

- 2 ripe avocados
- 1 can (5 ounces) tuna, drained
- 1/4 cup mayonnaise
- 1 tablespoon lemon juice
- 1 tablespoon fresh dill, chopped
- Salt and pepper to taste

Instructions:

1. Cut the avocados in half and remove the pits.
2. In a bowl, mix the tuna, mayonnaise, lemon juice, dill, salt, and pepper.
3. Scoop out a small amount of avocado flesh to create a larger cavity for the tuna salad.
4. Fill each avocado half with the tuna mixture.
5. Serve immediately.

Nutritional Values (per serving):

- Calories: 300
- Fat: 25g
- Carbohydrates: 10g
- Protein: 15g

Baked Salmon with Dill

Ingredients:

- 4 salmon fillets (about 6 ounces each)
- 2 tablespoons olive oil
- 2 tablespoons fresh dill, chopped
- 1 lemon, thinly sliced
- 1 teaspoon salt
- 1/2 teaspoon black pepper

Instructions:

1. Preheat your oven to 400°F (200°C).
2. Place the salmon fillets on a baking sheet lined with parchment paper.
3. Drizzle olive oil over the salmon fillets and rub it in to coat evenly.
4. Sprinkle the fillets with salt, black pepper, and chopped dill.
5. Arrange lemon slices on top of each fillet.
6. Bake in the preheated oven for 1215 minutes, or until the salmon is cooked through and flakes easily with a fork.
7. Serve hot, garnished with additional fresh dill if desired.

Nutritional Values (per serving):

- Calories: 280
- Fat: 18g
- Carbohydrates: 1g
- Protein: 28g

Grilled Chicken Breast with Herbs

Ingredients:

- 4 boneless, skinless chicken breasts
- 3 tablespoons olive oil
- 2 tablespoons fresh rosemary, chopped
- 2 tablespoons fresh thyme, chopped
- 1 teaspoon garlic powder
- 1 teaspoon salt
- 1/2 teaspoon black pepper

Instructions:

1. Preheat your grill to medium high heat.
2. In a small bowl, mix together olive oil, rosemary, thyme, garlic powder, salt, and black pepper.
3. Rub the herb mixture all over the chicken breasts, coating them evenly.
4. Place the chicken breasts on the grill and cook for 67 minutes per side, or until the internal temperature reaches 165°F

(75°C) and the chicken is no longer pink in the center.

5. Remove from the grill and let the chicken rest for a few minutes before serving.

Nutritional Values (per serving):

- Calories: 220
- Fat: 10g
- Carbohydrates: 1g
- Protein: 28g

Carrot Ginger Puree

Ingredients:

- 1 pound carrots, peeled and chopped
- 1 tablespoon fresh ginger, grated
- 2 cups vegetable broth or water
- 1 tablespoon olive oil
- 1/2 teaspoon salt
- 1/4 teaspoon black pepper

Instructions:

1. In a large pot, combine the chopped carrots, grated ginger, and vegetable broth (or water). Bring to a boil over medium high heat.
2. Reduce the heat and simmer for 1520 minutes, or until the carrots are very tender.
3. Use an immersion blender to puree the mixture until smooth.

Alternatively, transfer the mixture to a blender and puree until smooth.

4. Stir in the olive oil, salt, and pepper.
5. Serve warm.

Nutritional Values (per serving):

- Calories: 100
- Fat: 5g
- Carbohydrates: 12g
- Protein: 1g

Vegetable Stir Fry with Tofu

Ingredients:

- 1 block (14 ounces) firm tofu, drained and cubed
- 2 tablespoons soy sauce (gluten free if needed)
- 1 tablespoon sesame oil
- 1 red bell pepper, sliced
- 1 yellow bell pepper, sliced
- 1 cup broccoli florets
- 1 cup snap peas
- 2 cloves garlic, minced
- 1 tablespoon fresh ginger, grated
- 2 tablespoons olive oil

- Cooked rice or noodles for serving

Instructions:

1. In a small bowl, toss the tofu cubes with soy sauce and sesame oil. Let marinate for 10 minutes.
2. Heat 1 tablespoon of olive oil in a large skillet or wok over medium high heat. Add the marinated tofu and cook until golden brown on all sides. Remove from the skillet and set aside.
3. Add the remaining olive oil to the skillet. Add the garlic and ginger, and sauté until fragrant.
4. Add the bell peppers, broccoli, and snap peas to the skillet. Stir fry for 57 minutes, or until the vegetables are tender crisp.
5. Return the tofu to the skillet and toss to combine.
6. Serve hot over cooked rice or noodles.

Nutritional Values (per serving):

- Calories: 250
- Fat: 15g
- Carbohydrates: 20g
- Protein: 10g

Pulled Pork with Mashed Potatoes

Ingredients:

For the Pulled Pork:

- 2 pounds pork shoulder
- 1 cup barbecue sauce
- 1/2 cup apple cider vinegar
- 1/4 cup brown sugar
- 1 tablespoon paprika
- 1 tablespoon garlic powder
- 1 tablespoon onion powder
- Salt and pepper to taste

For the Mashed Potatoes:

- 4 large potatoes, peeled and cubed
- 1/2 cup milk
- 1/4 cup butter
- Salt and pepper to taste

Instructions:

1. Prepare the Pulled Pork:

- Preheat your oven to 300°F (150°C).
- In a small bowl, mix together the barbecue sauce, apple cider vinegar, brown sugar, paprika, garlic powder, onion powder, salt, and pepper.

- Place the pork shoulder in a roasting pan and pour the sauce mixture over it.
- Cover the pan with foil and bake for 45 hours, or until the pork is very tender and easily shredded with a fork.
- Shred the cooked pork and mix with the remaining sauce.

2. Prepare the Mashed Potatoes:

- In a large pot, boil the potatoes until tender, about 1520 minutes. Drain and return to the pot.
- Add the milk, butter, salt, and pepper to the potatoes. Mash until smooth and creamy.

3. Serve:

- Serve the shredded pork over the mashed potatoes. Enjoy!

Nutritional Values (per serving):

- Calories: 400
- Fat: 18g
- Carbohydrates: 35g
- Protein: 25g

Fennel and Orange Salad

Ingredients:

- 2 fennel bulbs, thinly sliced
- 2 oranges, peeled and segmented
- 1/4 red onion, thinly sliced
- 1/4 cup fresh mint leaves
- 3 tablespoons olive oil
- 1 tablespoon white wine vinegar
- Salt and pepper to taste

Instructions:

1. In a large bowl, combine the fennel, orange segments, red onion, and mint leaves.
2. In a small bowl, whisk together the olive oil, white wine vinegar, salt, and pepper.
3. Pour the dressing over the salad and toss to combine.
4. Serve chilled.

Nutritional Values (per serving):

- Calories: 120
- Fat: 8g
- Carbohydrates: 12g
- Protein: 1g

Egg Salad on Sourdough

Ingredients:

- 4 large eggs
- 1/4 cup mayonnaise
- 1 tablespoon Dijon mustard
- 1 tablespoon fresh dill, chopped
- Salt and pepper to taste
- 4 slices sourdough bread, toasted

Instructions:

1. Place the eggs in a pot and cover with water. Bring to a boil, then reduce heat and simmer for 10 minutes.
2. Drain and cool the eggs under cold running water. Peel and chop the eggs.
3. In a bowl, combine the chopped eggs, mayonnaise, Dijon mustard, dill, salt, and pepper.
4. Spread the egg salad onto the toasted sourdough bread.
5. Serve immediately.

Nutritional Values (per serving):

- Calories: 300
- Fat: 20g
- Carbohydrates: 20g
- Protein: 10g

Zucchini Noodles with Pesto

Ingredients:

- 4 medium zucchinis, spiralized
- 1/2 cup basil pesto (storebought or homemade)
- 1/4 cup cherry tomatoes, halved
- 2 tablespoons pine nuts
- 1 tablespoon olive oil
- Salt and pepper to taste

Instructions:

1. Heat the olive oil in a large skillet over medium heat.
2. Add the zucchini noodles and sauté for 23 minutes, or until just tender.
3. Remove from heat and toss with basil pesto, cherry tomatoes, and pine nuts.
4. Season with salt and pepper to taste.
5. Serve immediately.

Nutritional Values (per serving):

- Calories: 200
- Fat: 18g
- Carbohydrates: 8g
- Protein: 3g

Risotto with Asparagus

Ingredients:

- 1 cup Arborio rice
- 4 cups vegetable broth
- 1/2 cup dry white wine
- 1 bunch asparagus, trimmed and cut into 1inch pieces
- 1 small onion, finely chopped
- 2 cloves garlic, minced
- 1/4 cup Parmesan cheese, grated
- 2 tablespoons olive oil
- Salt and pepper to taste

Instructions:

1. In a saucepan, bring the vegetable broth to a simmer.
2. In a large pot, heat the olive oil over medium heat. Add the onion and garlic, and sauté until translucent.
3. Add the Arborio rice and cook, stirring constantly, for 23 minutes.
4. Pour in the white wine and cook until it is mostly absorbed.
5. Add the hot broth, one ladleful at a time, stirring frequently and allowing the liquid to be absorbed before adding more.
6. After 10 minutes, stir in the asparagus pieces.
7. Continue cooking and adding broth until the rice is creamy and tender, about 1820 minutes total.
8. Stir in the Parmesan cheese, and season with salt and pepper to taste.
9. Serve hot.

Nutritional Values (per serving):

- Calories: 350
- Fat: 10g
- Carbohydrates: 50g
- Protein: 10g

Potato Leek Soup

Ingredients:

- 4 large leeks, white and light green parts only, sliced
- 4 large potatoes, peeled and diced
- 4 cups vegetable broth
- 1 cup milk or cream
- 2 tablespoons butter
- 2 cloves garlic, minced

- Salt and pepper to taste

Instructions:

1. In a large pot, melt the butter over medium heat. Add the leeks and garlic, and sauté until soft, about 5 minutes.
2. Add the diced potatoes and vegetable broth. Bring to a boil, then reduce heat and simmer for 2025 minutes, or until the potatoes are tender.
3. Use an immersion blender to puree the soup until smooth. Alternatively, transfer the mixture to a blender and puree until smooth.
4. Stir in the milk or cream, and season with salt and pepper to taste.
5. Serve hot, optionally garnished with fresh herbs.

Nutritional Values (per serving):

- Calories: 250
- Fat: 10g
- Carbohydrates: 35g
- Protein: 5g

Baked Cod with Lemon and Herbs

Ingredients:

- 4 cod fillets (about 6 ounces each)
- 2 tablespoons olive oil
- 2 tablespoons fresh dill, chopped
- 1 lemon, thinly sliced
- 1 teaspoon salt
- 1/2 teaspoon black pepper

Instructions:

1. Preheat your oven to 400°F (200°C).
2. Place the cod fillets on a baking sheet lined with parchment paper.
3. Drizzle olive oil over the cod fillets and rub it in to coat evenly.
4. Sprinkle the fillets with salt, black pepper, and chopped dill.
5. Arrange lemon slices on top of each fillet.
6. Bake in the preheated oven for 1215 minutes, or until the cod is cooked through and flakes easily with a fork.
7. Serve hot, garnished with additional fresh dill if desired.

Nutritional Values (per serving):

- Calories: 180
- Fat: 10g
- Carbohydrates: 1g
- Protein: 20g

Shrimp and Rice Pilaf

Ingredients:

- 1 cup long grain rice
- 2 cups vegetable or chicken broth
- 1 pound shrimp, peeled and deveined
- 1 small onion, finely chopped
- 1 red bell pepper, diced
- 2 cloves garlic, minced
- 1 tablespoon olive oil
- 1/4 cup fresh parsley, chopped
- Salt and pepper to taste

Instructions:

1. In a medium pot, heat the olive oil over medium heat. Add the onion, red bell pepper, and garlic, and sauté until softened.
2. Add the rice and cook, stirring constantly, for 23 minutes.
3. Pour in the broth, bring to a boil, then reduce heat and simmer, covered, for 1520 minutes, or until the rice is tender and the liquid is absorbed.
4. In a separate skillet, cook the shrimp over medium heat until pink and opaque, about 23 minutes per side.
5. Stir the cooked shrimp and chopped parsley into the rice.
6. Season with salt and pepper to taste.
7. Serve hot.

Nutritional Values (per serving):

- Calories: 300
- Fat: 8g
- Carbohydrates: 35g
- Protein: 20g

Turkey and Spinach Meatballs

Ingredients:

- 1 pound ground turkey
- 1 cup fresh spinach, chopped
- 1/2 cup breadcrumbs
- 1/4 cup Parmesan cheese, grated
- 1 egg
- 2 cloves garlic, minced
- 1 teaspoon dried oregano
- Salt and pepper to taste
- 2 tablespoons olive oil

Instructions:

1. Preheat your oven to 375°F (190°C).

2. In a large bowl, combine the ground turkey, chopped spinach, breadcrumbs, Parmesan cheese, egg, garlic, oregano, salt, and pepper. Mix until well combined.
3. Form the mixture into meatballs, about 1 inch in diameter.
4. Heat the olive oil in a large skillet over medium heat. Add the meatballs and cook until browned on all sides.
5. Transfer the browned meatballs to a baking sheet and bake in the preheated oven for 1520 minutes, or until cooked through.
6. Serve hot.

Nutritional Values (per serving):

- Calories: 220
- Fat: 12g
- Carbohydrates: 10g
- Protein: 20g

Steamed Broccoli and Cauliflower

Ingredients:

- 1 head broccoli, cut into florets
- 1 head cauliflower, cut into florets
- 2 tablespoons olive oil
- Salt and pepper to taste
- Optional: lemon wedges for serving

Instructions:

1. Bring a large pot of water to a boil and place a steamer basket over it.
2. Add the broccoli and cauliflower florets to the steamer basket. Cover and steam for 57 minutes, or until tender but still crisp.
3. Remove from the steamer and transfer to a serving bowl.
4. Drizzle with olive oil and season with salt and pepper.
5. Serve with lemon wedges if desired.

Nutritional Values (per serving):

- Calories: 100
- Fat: 7g
- Carbohydrates: 8g
- Protein: 3g

Rice Congee

Ingredients:

- 1 cup long grain rice

- 8 cups water or chicken broth
- 1inch piece fresh ginger, sliced
- 2 green onions, sliced
- Salt and pepper to taste
- Optional toppings: shredded chicken, soy sauce, sesame oil, chopped cilantro

Instructions:

1. In a large pot, combine the rice, water or chicken broth, and ginger. Bring to a boil over high heat.
2. Reduce the heat to low and simmer, stirring occasionally, for about 11.5 hours, or until the rice has broken down and the congee is creamy.
3. Remove the ginger slices and season with salt and pepper to taste.
4. Serve hot with optional toppings like shredded chicken, soy sauce, sesame oil, or chopped cilantro.

Nutritional Values (per serving):

- Calories: 150
- Fat: 1g
- Carbohydrates: 30g
- Protein: 3g

Lentil Soup (without skins)

Ingredients:

- 1 cup red or yellow lentils, rinsed
- 1 large onion, chopped
- 2 carrots, diced
- 2 celery stalks, diced
- 3 cloves garlic, minced
- 1 teaspoon ground cumin
- 1 teaspoon ground turmeric
- 6 cups vegetable broth
- 2 tablespoons olive oil
- Salt and pepper to taste
- Fresh parsley for garnish

Instructions:

1. In a large pot, heat the olive oil over medium heat. Add the onion, carrots, and celery. Sauté until the vegetables are tender, about 5 minutes.
2. Add the garlic, cumin, and turmeric, and cook for another minute, stirring constantly.
3. Add the lentils and vegetable broth. Bring to a boil, then reduce heat and simmer for 2025 minutes, or until the lentils are tender.
4. Season with salt and pepper to taste.

5. Serve hot, garnished with fresh parsley.

Nutritional Values (per serving):

- Calories: 200
- Fat: 5g
- Carbohydrates: 30g
- Protein: 10g

Mashed Sweet Potatoes

Ingredients:

- 4 large sweet potatoes, peeled and cubed
- 1/2 cup milk (dairy or nondairy)
- 1/4 cup butter or dairy free alternative
- 1 tablespoon maple syrup or honey (optional)
- Salt and pepper to taste

Instructions:

1. In a large pot, bring water to a boil. Add the cubed sweet potatoes and cook until tender, about 1520 minutes. Drain and return to the pot.
2. Add the milk, butter, and maple syrup or honey (if using) to the sweet potatoes.

3. Mash until smooth and creamy.
4. Season with salt and pepper to taste.
5. Serve hot.

Nutritional Values (per serving):

- Calories: 200
- Fat: 7g
- Carbohydrates: 30g
- Protein: 2g

Chicken and Vegetable Kebabs

Ingredients:

- 1 -pound boneless, skinless chicken breasts, cut into 1inch cubes
- 1 red bell pepper, cut into 1inch pieces
- 1 yellow bell pepper, cut into 1inch pieces
- 1 zucchini, sliced into 1/2inch rounds
- 1 red onion, cut into wedges
- 2 tablespoons olive oil
- 2 tablespoons lemon juice
- 1 tablespoon fresh rosemary, chopped
- 1 tablespoon fresh thyme, chopped
- 2 cloves garlic, minced
- Salt and pepper to taste

Instructions:

1. In a large bowl, mix together olive oil, lemon juice, rosemary, thyme, garlic, salt, and pepper.
2. Add the chicken and vegetables to the bowl and toss to coat evenly. Let marinate for at least 30 minutes.
3. Preheat the grill to medium high heat.
4. Thread the chicken and vegetables onto skewers, alternating between chicken and vegetables.
5. Grill the kebabs for 1012 minutes, turning occasionally, until the chicken is cooked through and the vegetables are tender.
6. Serve hot.

Nutritional Values (per serving):

- Calories: 250
- Fat: 10g
- Carbohydrates: 10g
- Protein: 28g

Baked Beet and Carrot Salad

Ingredients:

- 3 medium beets, peeled and cut into wedges
- 3 large carrots, peeled and cut into sticks
- 2 tablespoons olive oil
- 1 tablespoon balsamic vinegar
- 1 tablespoon honey
- Salt and pepper to taste
- 1/4 cup crumbled goat cheese (optional)
- Fresh parsley, chopped, for garnish

Instructions:

1. Preheat the oven to 400°F (200°C).
2. In a large bowl, toss the beets and carrots with olive oil, balsamic vinegar, honey, salt, and pepper.
3. Spread the vegetables on a baking sheet lined with parchment paper.
4. Bake for 2530 minutes, or until the vegetables are tender and caramelized.
5. Transfer to a serving dish and sprinkle with goat cheese and fresh parsley if desired.
6. Serve warm or at room temperature.

Nutritional Values (per serving):

- Calories: 180
- Fat: 9g
- Carbohydrates: 25g

- Protein: 2g

Poached Pear Salad

Ingredients:

- 4 firm pears, peeled and halved
- 4 cups water
- 1/2 cup honey
- 1 cinnamon stick
- 1 star anise
- 4 cups mixed greens
- 1/4 cup walnuts, toasted
- 1/4 cup crumbled blue cheese (optional)
- 2 tablespoons balsamic glaze

Instructions:

1. In a large saucepan, combine water, honey, cinnamon stick, and star anise. Bring to a boil, then reduce heat and simmer.
2. Add the pear halves to the saucepan and simmer for 1520 minutes, or until the pears are tender.
3. Remove the pears from the poaching liquid and let cool.
4. Arrange mixed greens on a serving platter. Top with the poached pears, toasted walnuts, and crumbled blue cheese if using.
5. Drizzle with balsamic glaze before serving.

Nutritional Values (per serving):

- Calories: 220
- Fat: 10g
- Carbohydrates: 30g
- Protein: 3g

Dinner (25 Recipes)

Salmon Patties with Dill Sauce

Ingredients:

- 1 -pound fresh salmon, cooked and flaked (or canned salmon, drained and flaked)
- 1/2 cup breadcrumbs (gluten free if needed)
- 1 egg, beaten
- 2 tablespoons mayonnaise
- 1 tablespoon Dijon mustard
- 2 green onions, finely chopped
- 1 tablespoon fresh dill, chopped
- Salt and pepper to taste
- 2 tablespoons olive oil

For the Dill Sauce:

- 1/2 cup plain Greek yogurt
- 1 tablespoon fresh dill, chopped
- 1 tablespoon lemon juice
- Salt and pepper to taste

Instructions:

1. In a large bowl, combine the salmon, breadcrumbs, egg, mayonnaise, Dijon mustard, green onions, dill, salt, and pepper. Mix until well combined.
2. Form the mixture into patties (about 68 patties).
3. Heat the olive oil in a large skillet over medium heat. Cook the patties for 34 minutes on each side, or until golden brown and cooked through.
4. In a small bowl, mix together the Greek yogurt, dill, lemon juice, salt, and pepper to make the dill sauce.
5. Serve the salmon patties hot, topped with the dill sauce.

Nutritional Values (per serving):

- Calories: 300
- Fat: 20g
- Carbohydrates: 10g
- Protein: 20g

Roast Turkey with Carrots

Ingredients:

- 1 whole turkey (1214 pounds), thawed if frozen
- 1/4 cup olive oil
- 4 cloves garlic, minced
- 2 tablespoons fresh rosemary, chopped
- 2 tablespoons fresh thyme, chopped
- Salt and pepper to taste
- 1 -pound carrots, peeled and cut into large chunks
- 1 large onion, quartered
- 2 cups chicken broth

Instructions:

- Preheat your oven to 325°F (165°C).
- In a small bowl, mix together olive oil, garlic, rosemary, thyme, salt, and pepper.
- Rub the olive oil mixture all over the turkey, including under the skin and inside the cavity.
- Place the carrots and onion in the bottom of a large roasting pan. Pour the chicken broth over the vegetables.
- Place the turkey on a rack in the roasting pan, breast side up.
- Roast the turkey in the preheated oven, basting occasionally with the pan juices, for about 34 hours, or until the internal temperature reaches 165°F (75°C) in the thickest part of the thigh.
- Remove the turkey from the oven and let it rest for 20 minutes before carving.
- Serve the turkey with the roasted carrots and pan juices.

Nutritional Values (per serving):

- Calories: 350
- Fat: 20g
- Carbohydrates: 10g
- Protein: 30g

Baked Tilapia with Olive Tapenade

Ingredients:

- 4 tilapia fillets
- 2 tablespoons olive oil
- 1/2 teaspoon salt
- 1/4 teaspoon black pepper
- 1 cup olive tapenade (storebought or homemade)

For Homemade Olive Tapenade:

- 1 cup pitted black olives
- 2 cloves garlic
- 2 tablespoons capers
- 2 tablespoons olive oil
- 1 tablespoon lemon juice

Instructions:

1. Preheat your oven to 375°F (190°C).
2. Place the tilapia fillets on a baking sheet lined with parchment paper.
3. Drizzle the fillets with olive oil and season with salt and pepper.
4. Bake in the preheated oven for 1520 minutes, or until the fish is opaque and flakes easily with a fork.
5. To make the tapenade, combine olives, garlic, capers, olive oil, and lemon juice in a food processor. Pulse until finely chopped.
6. Serve the baked tilapia hot, topped with olive tapenade.

Nutritional Values (per serving):

- Calories: 250
- Fat: 15g
- Carbohydrates: 4g
- Protein: 20g

Lemon Herb Roasted Chicken

Ingredients:

- 1 whole chicken (about 4 pounds)
- 1/4 cup olive oil
- 3 cloves garlic, minced
- 2 tablespoons fresh lemon juice
- 1 tablespoon lemon zest
- 2 tablespoons fresh rosemary, chopped
- 2 tablespoons fresh thyme, chopped
- Salt and pepper to taste
- Lemon slices for garnish

Instructions:

1. Preheat your oven to 375°F (190°C).
2. In a small bowl, mix together olive oil, garlic, lemon juice, lemon zest, rosemary, thyme, salt, and pepper.
3. Rub the olive oil mixture all over the chicken, including under the skin and inside the cavity.
4. Place the chicken in a roasting pan and roast in the preheated oven for about 1 hour and 20 minutes, or until the internal temperature reaches 165°F (75°C).
5. Let the chicken rest for 10 minutes before carving.
6. Serve hot, garnished with lemon slices.

Nutritional Values (per serving):

- Calories: 300

- Fat: 20g
- Carbohydrates: 2g
- Protein: 25g

Creamy Polenta with Roasted Vegetables

Ingredients:

- For the Polenta:
- 1 cup polenta (coarse cornmeal)
- 4 cups water or vegetable broth
- 1/2 cup grated Parmesan cheese
- 2 tablespoons butter
- Salt and pepper to taste

For the Roasted Vegetables:

- 1 red bell pepper, chopped
- 1 yellow bell pepper, chopped
- 1 zucchini, sliced
- 1 red onion, chopped
- 2 tablespoons olive oil
- 1 teaspoon dried Italian herbs
- Salt and pepper to taste

Instructions:

1. Preheat your oven to 400°F (200°C).
2. Toss the chopped vegetables with olive oil, Italian herbs, salt, and pepper. Spread them out on a baking sheet.
3. Roast in the preheated oven for 2025 minutes, or until the vegetables are tender and slightly caramelized.
4. In a large saucepan, bring the water or vegetable broth to a boil. Gradually whisk in the polenta.
5. Reduce the heat and simmer, stirring frequently, until the polenta is thick and creamy, about 20 minutes.
6. Stir in the Parmesan cheese and butter. Season with salt and pepper to taste.
7. Serve the creamy polenta topped with the roasted vegetables.

Nutritional Values (per serving):

- Calories: 300
- Fat: 15g
- Carbohydrates: 35g
- Protein: 7g

Slow Cooker Beef Stew

Ingredients:

- 2 pounds beef stew meat, cut into 1-inch cubes
- 4 cups beef broth
- 4 carrots, sliced
- 4 potatoes, peeled and diced
- 1 large onion, chopped
- 3 cloves garlic, minced
- 1 teaspoon dried thyme
- 1 teaspoon dried rosemary
- 1 teaspoon salt
- 1/2 teaspoon black pepper
- 2 tablespoons tomato paste
- 2 tablespoons Worcestershire sauce
- 1/4 cup flour
- 1/4 cup water

Instructions:

1. Place the beef, carrots, potatoes, onion, and garlic into a slow cooker.
2. Add beef broth, thyme, rosemary, salt, pepper, tomato paste, and Worcestershire sauce. Stir to combine.
3. Cover and cook on low for 7-8 hours or on high for 4-5 hours until the meat and vegetables are tender.
4. In a small bowl, whisk together the flour and water until smooth. Stir into the stew and cook for an additional 30 minutes to thicken.
5. Serve hot.

Nutritional Values (per serving):

- Calories: 350
- Fat: 15g
- Carbohydrates: 30g
- Protein: 25g

Baked Haddock with Sweet Peppers

Ingredients:

- 4 haddock fillets
- 1 red bell pepper, sliced
- 1 yellow bell pepper, sliced
- 1 green bell pepper, sliced
- 2 tablespoons olive oil
- 1 teaspoon dried oregano
- 1 teaspoon dried basil
- Salt and pepper to taste
- Lemon wedges for serving

Instructions:

1. Preheat your oven to 375°F (190°C).
2. Place the haddock fillets on a baking sheet lined with parchment paper. Arrange the sliced bell peppers around the fillets.
3. Drizzle olive oil over the fish and peppers. Sprinkle with oregano, basil, salt, and pepper.
4. Bake in the preheated oven for 15-20 minutes, or until the fish

is opaque and flakes easily with a fork.

5. Serve hot with lemon wedges.

Nutritional Values (per serving):

- Calories: 200
- Fat: 10g
- Carbohydrates: 8g
- Protein: 20g

Pumpkin Risotto

Ingredients:

- 1 cup Arborio rice
- 4 cups vegetable broth, heated
- 1 cup pumpkin puree
- 1 small onion, finely chopped
- 2 cloves garlic, minced
- 1/2 cup dry white wine
- 1/2 cup grated Parmesan cheese
- 2 tablespoons butter
- 2 tablespoons olive oil
- 1 teaspoon dried sage
- Salt and pepper to taste

Instructions:

1. Heat the olive oil in a large saucepan over medium heat. Add the onion and cook until softened, about 5 minutes.
2. Add the garlic and Arborio rice, stirring to coat the rice with the oil.

3. Pour in the white wine and cook until absorbed.
4. Begin adding the heated vegetable broth, one ladleful at a time, stirring frequently and allowing each addition to be absorbed before adding the next.
5. When the rice is almost tender, stir in the pumpkin puree and dried sage. Continue to cook until the rice is creamy and fully cooked.
6. Stir in the butter and Parmesan cheese. Season with salt and pepper to taste.
7. Serve hot.

Nutritional Values (per serving):

- Calories: 350
- Fat: 15g
- Carbohydrates: 45g
- Protein: 10g

Vegetarian Chili

Ingredients:

- 1 tablespoon olive oil
- 1 large onion, chopped
- 3 cloves garlic, minced
- 2 bell peppers, chopped
- 2 carrots, chopped

- 2 zucchini, chopped
- 1 cup corn kernels
- 2 cans (15 ounces each) black beans, drained and rinsed
- 2 cans (15 ounces each) kidney beans, drained and rinsed
- 1 can (28 ounces) crushed tomatoes
- 2 tablespoons chili powder
- 1 tablespoon ground cumin
- 1 teaspoon paprika
- 1 teaspoon oregano
- Salt and pepper to taste

Instructions:

1. Heat the olive oil in a large pot over medium heat. Add the onion and garlic, and cook until softened, about 5 minutes.
2. Add the bell peppers, carrots, zucchini, and corn. Cook for another 5-7 minutes until the vegetables are tender.
3. Stir in the black beans, kidney beans, crushed tomatoes, chili powder, cumin, paprika, oregano, salt, and pepper.
4. Bring to a boil, then reduce the heat and simmer for 30 minutes, stirring occasionally.
5. Serve hot.

Nutritional Values (per serving):

- Calories: 250
- Fat: 5g
- Carbohydrates: 45g
- Protein: 12g

Stuffed Bell Peppers without Spices

Ingredients:

- 4 large bell peppers, tops cut off and seeds removed
- 1 cup cooked rice
- 1/2 -pound ground beef or turkey
- 1 cup canned diced tomatoes, drained
- 1/2 cup shredded mozzarella cheese
- Salt and pepper to taste

Instructions:

1. Preheat your oven to 375°F (190°C).
2. In a large skillet, cook the ground beef or turkey over medium heat until browned and cooked through. Drain any excess fat.
3. Add the cooked rice and diced tomatoes to the skillet. Season with salt and pepper. Mix until well combined.
4. Stuff each bell pepper with the meat and rice mixture, pressing down to fill completely.

5. Place the stuffed peppers in a baking dish and top with shredded mozzarella cheese.
6. Cover the dish with foil and bake in the preheated oven for 30 minutes. Remove the foil and bake for an additional 10 minutes, or until the cheese is melted and bubbly.
7. Serve hot.

Nutritional Values (per serving):

- Calories: 300
- Fat: 15g
- Carbohydrates: 20g
- Protein: 20g

Lamb Chops with Mint Pesto

Ingredients: For the Lamb Chops:

- 4 lamb chops
- 2 tablespoons olive oil
- Salt and pepper to taste
- For the Mint Pesto:
- 1 cup fresh mint leaves
- 1/4 cup pine nuts
- 1/4 cup grated Parmesan cheese
- 1 clove garlic
- 1/4 cup olive oil
- Salt and pepper to taste

Instructions:

1. Preheat a grill or grill pan over medium-high heat.
2. Brush the lamb chops with olive oil and season with salt and pepper.
3. Grill the lamb chops for 3-4 minutes per side, or until they reach your desired level of doneness.
4. To make the mint pesto, combine mint leaves, pine nuts, Parmesan cheese, garlic, and olive oil in a food processor. Blend until smooth. Season with salt and pepper to taste.
5. Serve the lamb chops hot, topped with mint pesto.

Nutritional Values (per serving):

- Calories: 400
- Fat: 30g
- Carbohydrates: 3g
- Protein: 25g

Simple Baked Tofu

Ingredients:

- 1 block (14 ounces) firm tofu, drained and pressed
- 2 tablespoons soy sauce (or tamari for gluten-free)
- 1 tablespoon olive oil

Instructions:

1. Preheat your oven to 375°F (190°C).
2. Cut the tofu into 1-inch cubes and place in a bowl.
3. Drizzle with soy sauce and olive oil. Toss to coat evenly.
4. Spread the tofu cubes on a baking sheet lined with parchment paper.
5. Bake in the preheated oven for 25-30 minutes, or until the tofu is golden brown and crispy on the edges.
6. Serve hot.

Nutritional Values (per serving):

- Calories: 200
- Fat: 12g
- Carbohydrates: 6g
- Protein: 16g

Roasted Duck with Orange Sauce

Ingredients: For the Duck:

- 1 whole duck (about 4-5 pounds)
- Salt and pepper to taste
- For the Orange Sauce:
- 1 cup fresh orange juice
- 1/4 cup honey
- 2 tablespoons soy sauce
- 1 tablespoon cornstarch mixed with 2 tablespoons water

Instructions:

1. Preheat your oven to 350°F (175°C).
2. Pat the duck dry with paper towels and season generously with salt and pepper.
3. Place the duck on a rack in a roasting pan.
4. Roast in the preheated oven for about 2 hours, or until the internal temperature reaches 165°F (75°C).
5. To make the orange sauce, combine orange juice, honey, and soy sauce in a small saucepan. Bring to a simmer over medium heat.
6. Stir in the cornstarch mixture and cook until the sauce thickens.
7. Serve the roasted duck hot, with orange sauce drizzled over the top.

Nutritional Values (per serving):

- Calories: 450
- Fat: 30g
- Carbohydrates: 20g
- Protein: 25g

Spaghetti Squash with Marinara Sauce

Ingredients:

- 1 large spaghetti squash
- 2 cups marinara sauce (store-bought or homemade)
- 1/4 cup grated Parmesan cheese
- 2 tablespoons olive oil
- Salt and pepper to taste

Instructions:

1. Preheat your oven to 375°F (190°C).
2. Cut the spaghetti squash in half lengthwise and remove the seeds.
3. Drizzle with olive oil and season with salt and pepper.
4. Place the squash halves cut-side down on a baking sheet. Roast in the preheated oven for 40-45 minutes, or until tender.
5. Using a fork, scrape the flesh of the squash to create spaghetti-like strands.
6. Heat the marinara sauce in a saucepan over medium heat.
7. Serve the spaghetti squash topped with marinara sauce and grated Parmesan cheese.

Nutritional Values (per serving):

- Calories: 200
- Fat: 10g
- Carbohydrates: 25g
- Protein: 6g

Turkey Meatloaf

Ingredients:

- 1 pound ground turkey
- 1/2 cup breadcrumbs (gluten-free if needed)
- 1/4 cup milk (dairy or non-dairy)
- 1 egg, beaten
- 1 small onion, finely chopped
- 2 cloves garlic, minced
- 2 tablespoons ketchup
- 1 tablespoon Worcestershire sauce
- 1 teaspoon dried thyme
- Salt and pepper to taste

Instructions:

1. Preheat your oven to 375°F (190°C).
2. In a large bowl, combine ground turkey, breadcrumbs, milk, egg, onion, garlic, ketchup, Worcestershire sauce, thyme, salt, and pepper. Mix until well combined.

3. Shape the mixture into a loaf and place it in a baking dish.
4. Bake in the preheated oven for 45-50 minutes, or until the internal temperature reaches 165°F (75°C).
5. Let the meatloaf rest for 10 minutes before slicing.
6. Serve hot.

Nutritional Values (per serving):

- Calories: 250
- Fat: 12g
- Carbohydrates: 15g
- Protein: 20g
- Health Benefits:

Vegetable Paella

Ingredients:

- 1 cup Arborio rice
- 1 red bell pepper, sliced
- 1 yellow bell pepper, sliced
- 1 zucchini, sliced
- 1 cup green beans, trimmed
- 1 cup cherry tomatoes, halved
- 4 cups vegetable broth
- 1/2 teaspoon saffron threads (optional)
- 2 cloves garlic, minced
- 1 onion, chopped
- 2 tablespoons olive oil
- Salt and pepper to taste
- Fresh parsley for garnish

Instructions:

1. Heat the olive oil in a large skillet or paella pan over medium heat. Add the onion and garlic, cooking until softened, about 5 minutes.
2. Add the Arborio rice and stir to coat with the oil.
3. Pour in the vegetable broth and saffron threads, if using. Bring to a boil, then reduce the heat and simmer.
4. Add the bell peppers, zucchini, green beans, and cherry tomatoes. Stir to combine.
5. Cook for about 20 minutes, or until the rice is tender and the liquid is absorbed.
6. Season with salt and pepper to taste.
7. Serve hot, garnished with fresh parsley.

Nutritional Values (per serving):

- Calories: 250
- Fat: 8g
- Carbohydrates: 38g
- Protein: 5g
- Health Benefits:

Fish Tacos with Cabbage Slaw

Ingredients: For the Fish:

- 1- pound white fish fillets (such as cod or tilapia)
- 2 tablespoons olive oil
- 1 tablespoon lime juice
- Salt and pepper to taste
- For the Cabbage Slaw:
- 2 cups shredded cabbage
- ¼ cup shredded carrots
- 2 tablespoons chopped cilantro
- 2 tablespoons lime juice
- 1 tablespoon olive oil
- Salt and pepper to taste
- To Serve:
- 8 small corn tortillas
- Lime wedges

Instructions:

1. Preheat your grill or grill pan over medium-high heat.
2. Brush the fish fillets with olive oil and lime juice. Season with salt and pepper.
3. Grill the fish for about 3-4 minutes per side, or until cooked through and flaky.
4. In a large bowl, combine cabbage, carrots, cilantro, lime juice, olive oil, salt, and pepper to make the slaw. Toss to coat.
5. Warm the tortillas on the grill or in a dry skillet.
6. To assemble the tacos, place grilled fish on each tortilla and top with cabbage slaw. Serve with lime wedges.

Nutritional Values (per serving):

- Calories: 200
- Fat: 10g
- Carbohydrates: 20g
- Protein: 15g

Chicken Pot Pie without Onion/Garlic

Ingredients:

- 1 -pound boneless, skinless chicken breasts, cubed
- 1 cup frozen peas and carrots
- 1 cup diced potatoes
- 1 cup chicken broth
- 1 cup milk (dairy or non-dairy)
- 1/4 cup all-purpose flour
- 1/4 cup butter
- 1 teaspoon dried thyme
- Salt and pepper to taste
- 1 sheet puff pastry, thawed

Instructions:

1. Preheat your oven to 400°F (200°C).

2. In a large pot, cook the diced potatoes until tender. Drain and set aside.
3. In a large skillet, melt the butter over medium heat. Add the chicken and cook until no longer pink.
4. Stir in the flour and cook for 1-2 minutes.
5. Gradually add the chicken broth and milk, stirring until the mixture thickens.
6. Add the frozen peas and carrots, cooked potatoes, thyme, salt, and pepper. Cook until the mixture is heated through.
7. Transfer the chicken mixture to a baking dish. Top with the puff pastry, trimming any excess.
8. Bake in the preheated oven for 20-25 minutes, or until the pastry is golden brown.
9. Serve hot.

Nutritional Values (per serving):

- Calories: 350
- Fat: 20g
- Carbohydrates: 25g
- Protein: 20g

Stuffed Acorn Squash

Ingredients:

- 2 medium acorn squashes, halved and seeds removed
- 1 cup cooked quinoa
- 1/2 cup dried cranberries
- 1/4 cup chopped pecans
- 1/4 cup feta cheese, crumbled
- 2 tablespoons olive oil
- Salt and pepper to taste

Instructions:

1. Preheat your oven to 375°F (190°C).
2. Drizzle the acorn squash halves with olive oil and season with salt and pepper. Place them cut-side down on a baking sheet and roast for 30-35 minutes, or until tender.
3. In a large bowl, combine cooked quinoa, dried cranberries, chopped pecans, and feta cheese. Season with salt and pepper.
4. Stuff each acorn squash half with the quinoa mixture.
5. Return to the oven and bake for an additional 10 minutes.
6. Serve hot.

Nutritional Values (per serving):

- Calories: 300
- Fat: 15g
- Carbohydrates: 40g
- Protein: 8g

Basil Chicken over Rice

Ingredients:

- 1- pound boneless, skinless chicken breasts, sliced
- 1 cup fresh basil leaves
- 2 cloves garlic, minced
- 1/4 cup soy sauce (or tamari for gluten-free)
- 2 tablespoons olive oil
- 2 cups cooked jasmine rice

Instructions:

1. Heat the olive oil in a large skillet over medium-high heat.
2. Add the sliced chicken and cook until browned and cooked through.
3. Add the garlic and cook for an additional minute.
4. Stir in the soy sauce and fresh basil leaves. Cook until the basil is wilted.
5. Serve the basil chicken over cooked jasmine rice.

Nutritional Values (per serving):

- Calories: 350

- Fat: 12g
- Carbohydrates: 30g
- Protein: 25g

Eggplant Parmesan without Seeds

Ingredients:

- 2 large eggplants, peeled and sliced into 1/2-inch rounds
- 1 teaspoon salt
- 1 cup all-purpose flour (gluten-free if needed)
- 2 eggs, beaten
- 1 cup breadcrumbs (gluten-free if needed)
- 2 cups marinara sauce
- 2 cups shredded mozzarella cheese
- 1/2 cup grated Parmesan cheese
- 1/4 cup fresh basil leaves, chopped
- Olive oil for frying

Instructions:

1. Preheat your oven to 375°F (190°C).
2. Sprinkle the eggplant slices with salt and let them sit for 30 minutes to draw out excess moisture. Pat dry with paper towels.

3. Dredge each eggplant slice in flour, dip in beaten eggs, and coat with breadcrumbs.
4. Heat olive oil in a large skillet over medium heat. Fry the eggplant slices until golden brown on both sides. Drain on paper towels.
5. In a baking dish, spread a thin layer of marinara sauce. Layer half of the eggplant slices, top with more marinara sauce, mozzarella, and Parmesan cheese. Repeat with remaining ingredients.
6. Bake in the preheated oven for 20-25 minutes, or until the cheese is bubbly and golden brown.
7. Garnish with fresh basil before serving.

Nutritional Values (per serving):

- Calories: 350
- Fat: 18g
- Carbohydrates: 32g
- Protein: 14g

Portobello Mushroom Steaks

Ingredients:

- 4 large portobello mushrooms, stems removed
- 1/4 cup balsamic vinegar
- 2 tablespoons olive oil
- 2 cloves garlic, minced
- 1 teaspoon dried thyme
- Salt and pepper to taste

Instructions:

1. In a small bowl, whisk together balsamic vinegar, olive oil, garlic, thyme, salt, and pepper.
2. Place the portobello mushrooms in a shallow dish and pour the marinade over them. Let marinate for at least 30 minutes.
3. Preheat your grill to medium-high heat.
4. Grill the mushrooms for 5-7 minutes on each side, or until tender and slightly charred.
5. Serve hot, garnished with fresh herbs if desired.

Nutritional Values (per serving):

- Calories: 100
- Fat: 7g
- Carbohydrates: 8g
- Protein: 3g

Turkey and Rice Casserole

Ingredients:

- 1 pound ground turkey
- 1 cup long-grain white rice
- 2 cups chicken broth
- 1 cup frozen peas and carrots
- 1 small onion, chopped
- 2 cloves garlic, minced
- 1 teaspoon dried thyme
- 1 teaspoon salt
- 1/2 teaspoon black pepper
- 1 cup shredded cheddar cheese
- 2 tablespoons olive oil

Instructions:

1. Preheat your oven to 375°F (190°C).
2. In a large skillet, heat olive oil over medium heat. Add the onion and garlic, and cook until softened, about 5 minutes.
3. Add the ground turkey and cook until browned, breaking it up with a spoon.
4. Stir in the rice, chicken broth, peas and carrots, thyme, salt, and pepper. Bring to a boil, then reduce heat and simmer for 10 minutes.
5. Transfer the mixture to a greased baking dish. Top with shredded cheddar cheese.
6. Bake in the preheated oven for 25-30 minutes, or until the cheese is melted and bubbly.
7. Serve hot.

Nutritional Values (per serving):

- Calories: 350
- Fat: 15g
- Carbohydrates: 30g
- Protein: 25g

Shepherd's Pie with Lentils

Ingredients:

- 1 cup green or brown lentils, rinsed and drained
- 2 cups vegetable broth
- 1 onion, chopped
- 2 cloves garlic, minced
- 2 carrots, diced
- 1 cup frozen peas
- 1 cup corn kernels
- 2 tablespoons tomato paste
- 1 teaspoon dried thyme
- 1 teaspoon dried rosemary
- Salt and pepper to taste
- 4 cups mashed potatoes (prepared with milk and butter)
- 2 tablespoons olive oil

Instructions:

1. Preheat your oven to 375°F (190°C).
2. In a large skillet, heat olive oil over medium heat. Add the onion, garlic, and carrots. Cook until softened, about 5 minutes.

3. Add the lentils, vegetable broth, tomato paste, thyme, rosemary, salt, and pepper. Bring to a boil, then reduce heat and simmer for 20-25 minutes, or until the lentils are tender and most of the liquid is absorbed.
4. Stir in the peas and corn, and cook for another 5 minutes.
5. Transfer the lentil mixture to a greased baking dish. Spread the mashed potatoes evenly over the top.
6. Bake in the preheated oven for 25-30 minutes, or until the top is golden brown.
7. Serve hot.

Nutritional Values (per serving):

- Calories: 300
- Fat: 10g
- Carbohydrates: 45g
- Protein: 10g

Soft Shell Crab with Ginger Aioli

Ingredients: *For the Soft- Shell Crab:*

- 8 soft shell crabs, cleaned and patted dry
- 1 cup all -purpose flour
- 1 teaspoon salt
- 1/2 teaspoon black pepper
- 1/2 teaspoon paprika
- 2 eggs, beaten
- 1/2 cup milk
- 1 cup panko breadcrumbs
- 1/2 cup vegetable oil for frying
- Lemon wedges for serving

For the Ginger Aioli:

- 1/2 cup mayonnaise
- 1 tablespoon fresh ginger, finely grated
- 1 clove garlic, minced
- 1 tablespoon lemon juice
- Salt and pepper to taste

Instructions:

1. Prepare the Ginger Aioli:

- In a small bowl, combine the mayonnaise, grated ginger, minced garlic, lemon juice, salt, and pepper. Mix well until smooth.
- Cover and refrigerate until ready to serve.

2. Prepare the Soft -Shell Crab:

- In a shallow dish, mix the flour, salt, black pepper, and paprika.
- In another shallow dish, whisk together the beaten eggs and milk.
- In a third shallow dish, place the panko breadcrumbs.

- Dredge each soft -shell crab in the flour mixture, shaking off any excess.
- Dip the crab into the egg mixture, then coat with panko breadcrumbs, pressing gently to adhere.

3. Fry the Crabs:

- In a large skillet, heat the vegetable oil over medium high heat until shimmering.
- Fry the crabs in batches, cooking for about 34 minutes per side, or until golden brown and crispy.
- Transfer the fried crabs to a paper towellined plate to drain excess oil.

4. Serve:

- Serve the soft- shell crabs hot, with lemon wedges on the side.
- Accompany with the ginger aioli for dipping.

Nutritional Values (per serving):

- Calories: 400
- Fat: 25g
- Carbohydrates: 30g
- Protein: 15g

Snacks (25 Recipes)

Rice Cakes with Almond Butter

Ingredients:

- 4 rice cakes (plain or lightly salted)
- 1/2 cup almond butter
- Optional toppings: banana slices, chia seeds, or a drizzle of honey

Instructions:

1. Spread a generous layer of almond butter over each rice cake.
2. Add optional toppings such as banana slices, chia seeds, or a drizzle of honey for added flavor and nutrition.
3. Serve immediately.

Nutritional Values (per serving of 2 rice cakes with almond butter):

- Calories: 220
- Fat: 14g
- Carbohydrates: 22g
- Protein: 6g

Homemade Apple Sauce

Ingredients:

- 6 large apples (such as Granny Smith, Fuji, or Honeycrisp), peeled, cored, and chopped
- 1/2 cup water
- 1/4 cup sugar (optional, adjust to taste)
- 1 teaspoon ground cinnamon
- 1 tablespoon lemon juice

Instructions:

1. In a large pot, combine the chopped apples, water, sugar (if using), and ground cinnamon.
2. Bring to a boil over mediumhigh heat, then reduce the heat to low.
3. Cover and simmer for about 2030 minutes, or until the apples are very soft.
4. Remove from heat and stir in the lemon juice.
5. Use an immersion blender to blend the apples to your desired consistency (smooth or chunky). Alternatively, you can mash the apples with a fork or

potato masher for a chunkier texture.

6. Let the apple sauce cool before transferring it to an airtight container. Refrigerate until ready to serve.

Nutritional Values (per serving):

- Calories: 100
- Fat: 0g
- Carbohydrates: 26g
- Protein: 0g

Baked Plantain Chips

Ingredients:

- 2 large green plantains
- 2 tablespoons olive oil or coconut oil
- 1/2 teaspoon salt
- Optional: 1/2 teaspoon smoked paprika, garlic powder, or chili powder for added flavor

Instructions:

1. Preheat your oven to 375°F (190°C) and line a baking sheet with parchment paper.
2. Peel the plantains and slice them thinly (about 1/8 inch thick) using a mandoline or a sharp knife.
3. In a large bowl, toss the plantain slices with olive oil and salt until evenly coated. Add any optional seasonings if desired.
4. Arrange the plantain slices in a single layer on the prepared baking sheet.
5. Bake in the preheated oven for 1520 minutes, flipping the chips halfway through, until they are golden brown and crispy.
6. Remove from the oven and let cool on the baking sheet. The chips will continue to crisp up as they cool.
7. Serve immediately or store in an airtight container for up to a week.

Nutritional Values (per serving):

- Calories: 150
- Fat: 7g
- Carbohydrates: 21g
- Protein: 1g

Mashed Avocado with Salt

Ingredients:

- 2 ripe avocados
- 1/2 teaspoon salt (or to taste)
- Optional: a squeeze of lime juice

Instructions:

1. Cut the avocados in half, remove the pits, and scoop the flesh into a bowl.
2. Mash the avocados with a fork until you reach your desired consistency (smooth or chunky).
3. Stir in the salt and mix well.
4. If using, add a squeeze of lime juice for added flavor and to help prevent browning.
5. Serve immediately as a spread on toast, a dip, or a side dish.

Nutritional Values (per serving):

- Calories: 160
- Fat: 15g
- Carbohydrates: 9g
- Protein: 2g

Yogurt with Maple Syrup

Ingredients:

- 1 cup plain Greek yogurt (or any yogurt of choice)
- 12 tablespoons maple syrup (adjust to taste)
- Optional toppings: fresh berries, granola, or nuts

Instructions:

1. Place the yogurt in a bowl.
2. Drizzle the maple syrup over the yogurt.
3. Stir gently to combine.
4. Add optional toppings such as fresh berries, granola, or nuts for added texture and flavor.
5. Serve immediately.

Nutritional Values (per serving):

- Calories: 180
- Fat: 4g
- Carbohydrates: 25g
- Protein: 12g

Cucumber Slices with Hummus

Ingredients:

- 1 large cucumber, sliced into rounds
- 1 cup hummus (storebought or homemade)

Instructions:

1. Wash the cucumber thoroughly and slice it into rounds.
2. Arrange the cucumber slices on a serving platter.
3. Serve the cucumber slices with hummus on the side for dipping.
4. Enjoy as a healthy snack or appetizer.

Nutritional Values (per serving):

- Calories: 150
- Fat: 8g
- Carbohydrates: 14g
- Protein: 6g

Roasted Chickpeas (Low-Salt)

Ingredients:

- 1 can (15 ounces) chickpeas, drained and rinsed
- 1 tablespoon olive oil
- 1/2 teaspoon salt
- Optional: 1/2 teaspoon paprika, garlic powder, or cumin for extra flavor

Instructions:

1. Preheat your oven to 400°F (200°C).
2. Pat the chickpeas dry with a paper towel to remove excess moisture.
3. In a bowl, toss the chickpeas with olive oil, salt, and any optional spices.
4. Spread the chickpeas on a baking sheet in a single layer.
5. Roast in the preheated oven for 2030 minutes, stirring occasionally, until the chickpeas are crispy.
6. Remove from the oven and let cool before serving.

Nutritional Values (per serving):

- Calories: 150
- Fat: 6g
- Carbohydrates: 20g
- Protein: 6g

Carrot Sticks with Tahini Dip

Ingredients:

- For the Carrot Sticks:
- 4 large carrots, peeled and cut into sticks

For the Tahini Dip:

- 1/4 cup tahini
- 2 tablespoons lemon juice
- 1 clove garlic, minced
- 23 tablespoons water (to reach desired consistency)
- Salt to taste

Instructions:

1. In a bowl, whisk together the tahini, lemon juice, minced garlic, and salt. Gradually add water until the dip reaches your desired consistency.
2. Arrange the carrot sticks on a serving platter.
3. Serve the carrot sticks with the tahini dip.

Nutritional Values (per serving):

- Calories: 120
- Fat: 9g
- Carbohydrates: 10g
- Protein: 3g

Baked Peach Slices

Ingredients:

- 4 ripe peaches, sliced
- 1 tablespoon honey or maple syrup
- 1 teaspoon cinnamon

Instructions:

1. Preheat your oven to 375°F (190°C).

2. Arrange the peach slices on a baking sheet lined with parchment paper.
3. Drizzle the peaches with honey or maple syrup and sprinkle with cinnamon.
4. Bake in the preheated oven for 1520 minutes, or until the peaches are tender and caramelized.
5. Serve warm.

Nutritional Values (per serving):

- Calories: 100
- Fat: 0g
- Carbohydrates: 25g
- Protein: 1g

Rice Pudding

Ingredients:

- 1/2 cup white rice
- 4 cups milk (dairy or nondairy)
- 1/4 cup sugar
- 1 teaspoon vanilla extract
- 1/2 teaspoon ground cinnamon

Instructions:

1. In a large saucepan, combine the rice, milk, and sugar.
2. Bring to a boil over medium high heat, then reduce the heat to low and simmer, stirring

frequently, for 3040 minutes, or until the rice is tender and the pudding is thickened.

3. Stir in the vanilla extract and ground cinnamon.
4. Serve warm or chilled.

Nutritional Values (per serving):

- Calories: 200
- Fat: 5g
- Carbohydrates: 35g
- Protein: 6g

Banana Bread (Low-Fiber)

Ingredients:

- 2 ripe bananas, mashed
- 1/2 cup sugar
- 1/4 cup butter, melted
- 1 egg
- 1 teaspoon vanilla extract
- 1 1/2 cups all-purpose flour
- 1 teaspoon baking soda
- 1/2 teaspoon salt

Instructions:

1. Preheat your oven to 350°F (175°C). Grease a loaf pan.
2. In a large bowl, mix the mashed bananas, sugar, melted butter, egg, and vanilla extract.
3. In another bowl, whisk together the flour, baking soda, and salt.

4. Gradually add the dry ingredients to the banana mixture, stirring until just combined.
5. Pour the batter into the prepared loaf pan.
6. Bake in the preheated oven for 6070 minutes, or until a toothpick inserted into the center comes out clean.
7. Let cool before slicing.

Nutritional Values (per serving):

- Calories: 180
- Fat: 6g
- Carbohydrates: 30g
- Protein: 3g

Pumpkin Seeds (Peeled)

Ingredients:

- 1 cup raw pumpkin seeds (pepitas)
- 1 teaspoon olive oil
- 1/2 teaspoon salt
- Optional: 1/2 teaspoon smoked paprika or chili powder

Instructions:

1. Preheat your oven to 350°F (175°C).

2. In a bowl, toss the pumpkin seeds with olive oil, salt, and optional spices.
3. Spread the seeds in a single layer on a baking sheet.
4. Bake in the preheated oven for 1015 minutes, or until golden brown, stirring occasionally.
5. Let cool before serving.

Nutritional Values (per serving):

- Calories: 180
- Fat: 14g
- Carbohydrates: 4g
- Protein: 9g

Smooth Nut Butter Balls

Ingredients:

- 1 cup nut butter (such as almond or peanut butter)
- 1/4 cup honey or maple syrup
- 1/2 cup rolled oats (gluten free if needed)
- 1/4 cup unsweetened shredded coconut

Instructions:

1. In a bowl, combine the nut butter, honey or maple syrup, rolled oats, and shredded coconut. Mix until well combined.

2. Roll the mixture into small balls, about 1 inch in diameter.
3. Place the balls on a baking sheet lined with parchment paper.
4. Refrigerate for at least 30 minutes before serving.

Nutritional Values (per serving):

- Calories: 150
- Fat: 10g
- Carbohydrates: 15g
- Protein: 4g

Coconut Water Popsicles

Ingredients:

- 2 cups coconut water
- 1 cup diced fresh fruit (such as strawberries, mango, or kiwi)

Instructions:

1. In a bowl, combine the coconut water and diced fresh fruit.
2. Pour the mixture into popsicle molds.
3. Insert popsicle sticks and freeze for at least 4 hours, or until solid.

4. To serve, run the molds under warm water to release the popsicles.

Nutritional Values (per serving):

- Calories: 50
- Fat: 0g
- Carbohydrates: 12g
- Protein: 0g

Sliced Melon

Ingredients:

- 1 large melon (such as cantaloupe, honeydew, or watermelon)

Instructions:

1. Cut the melon in half and remove the seeds.
2. Slice the melon into wedges or cubes.
3. Arrange the melon slices on a serving platter.
4. Serve chilled.

Nutritional Values (per serving):

- Calories: 60
- Fat: 0g
- Carbohydrates: 15g
- Protein: 1g

Steamed Edamame (Peeled)

Ingredients:

- 2 cups edamame (fresh or frozen)
- 1/2 teaspoon salt

Instructions:

1. Bring a pot of water to a boil. Add the edamame and cook for 57 minutes, or until tender.
2. Drain the edamame and sprinkle with salt.
3. Serve warm or chilled.

Nutritional Values (per serving):

- Calories: 120
- Fat: 5g
- Carbohydrates: 10g
- Protein: 12g

Soft Baked Pears

Ingredients:

- 4 ripe pears, halved and cored
- 2 tablespoons honey or maple syrup
- 1 teaspoon ground cinnamon

Instructions:

1. Preheat your oven to 350°F (175°C).
2. Arrange the pear halves in a baking dish.
3. Drizzle the pears with honey or maple syrup and sprinkle with cinnamon.
4. Bake in the preheated oven for 2025 minutes, or until the pears are tender.
5. Serve warm.

Nutritional Values (per serving):

- Calories: 100
- Fat: 0g
- Carbohydrates: 26g
- Protein: 0g

Non-dairy Chocolate Pudding

Ingredients:

- 1 can (14 ounces) coconut milk
- 1/4 cup cocoa powder
- 1/4 cup cornstarch
- 1/4 cup maple syrup or honey
- 1 teaspoon vanilla extract
- Pinch of salt

Instructions:

1. In a saucepan, whisk together the coconut milk, cocoa powder, cornstarch, maple syrup or honey, vanilla extract, and salt.
2. Cook over medium heat, stirring constantly, until the mixture thickens and comes to a boil.
3. Remove from heat and let cool slightly.
4. Pour the pudding into individual serving bowls.
5. Refrigerate for at least 2 hours before serving.

Nutritional Values (per serving):

- Calories: 200
- Fat: 12g
- Carbohydrates: 25g
- Protein: 2g

Gelatin with Fruit Juice

Ingredients:

- 2 cups 100% fruit juice (such as apple, grape, or orange)
- 2 tablespoons unflavored gelatin powder
- 1 tablespoon honey or sugar (optional)

Instructions:

1. Pour 1 cup of fruit juice into a bowl. Sprinkle the gelatin

powder over the juice and let it sit for a few minutes to bloom.
2. In a saucepan, heat the remaining 1 cup of fruit juice until warm but not boiling. Stir in the honey or sugar if using.
3. Pour the warm juice into the bowl with the gelatin and stir until the gelatin is fully dissolved.
4. Pour the mixture into molds or a shallow dish.
5. Refrigerate for at least 4 hours, or until set.
6. Serve chilled.

Nutritional Values (per serving):

- Calories: 80
- Fat: 0g
- Carbohydrates: 18g
- Protein: 2g

Soft Baked Apple Slices

Ingredients:

- 4 large apples, peeled, cored, and sliced
- 2 tablespoons honey or maple syrup
- 1 teaspoon ground cinnamon

Instructions:

1. Preheat your oven to 350°F (175°C).
2. Arrange the apple slices in a baking dish.
3. Drizzle with honey or maple syrup and sprinkle with cinnamon.
4. Bake in the preheated oven for 2025 minutes, or until the apples are tender.
5. Serve warm.

Nutritional Values (per serving):

- Calories: 100
- Fat: 0g
- Carbohydrates: 26g
- Protein: 0g

Guacamole

Ingredients:

- 3 ripe avocados
- 1 small onion, finely chopped
- 1 medium tomato, diced
- 1 clove garlic, minced
- 1 jalapeno, seeded and minced (optional)
- 1/4 cup fresh cilantro, chopped
- Juice of 1 lime
- 1/2 teaspoon salt

Instructions:

1. Cut the avocados in half, remove the pits, and scoop the flesh into a bowl.
2. Mash the avocados with a fork until you reach your desired consistency.
3. Add the onion, tomato, garlic, jalapeno (if using), cilantro, lime juice, and salt.
4. Stir well to combine.
5. Serve immediately with tortilla chips, vegetable sticks, or as a topping for tacos.

Nutritional Values (per serving):

- Calories: 200
- Fat: 18g
- Carbohydrates: 12g
- Protein: 2g

Squash Soup

Ingredients:

- 1 large butternut squash, peeled, seeded, and cubed
- 1 large onion, chopped
- 3 cloves garlic, minced
- 4 cups vegetable broth
- 2 tablespoons olive oil
- 1 teaspoon ground cumin
- 1/2 teaspoon ground nutmeg
- Salt and pepper to taste

- Optional: 1/2 cup coconut milk for added creaminess

Instructions:

1. In a large pot, heat the olive oil over medium heat. Add the chopped onion and garlic, and cook until softened, about 5 minutes.
2. Add the cubed butternut squash, vegetable broth, cumin, nutmeg, salt, and pepper.
3. Bring to a boil, then reduce the heat and simmer for 2025 minutes, or until the squash is tender.
4. Use an immersion blender to puree the soup until smooth. Alternatively, transfer the soup to a blender in batches and blend until smooth.
5. If using, stir in the coconut milk and heat through.
6. Serve hot, garnished with fresh herbs if desired.

Nutritional Values (per serving):

- Calories: 150
- Fat: 7g
- Carbohydrates: 20g
- Protein: 2g

Baked Potato Wedges

Ingredients:

- 4 large potatoes, washed and cut into wedges
- 2 tablespoons olive oil
- 1 teaspoon garlic powder
- 1 teaspoon paprika
- 1/2 teaspoon salt
- 1/2 teaspoon black pepper
- Optional: chopped fresh parsley for garnish

Instructions:

1. Preheat your oven to 425°F (220°C).
2. In a large bowl, toss the potato wedges with olive oil, garlic powder, paprika, salt, and black pepper until evenly coated.
3. Spread the potato wedges in a single layer on a baking sheet lined with parchment paper.
4. Bake in the preheated oven for 2530 minutes, turning once, until golden brown and crispy.
5. Remove from the oven and sprinkle with fresh parsley if desired.
6. Serve hot.

Nutritional Values (per serving):

- Calories: 200
- Fat: 7g
- Carbohydrates: 32g
- Protein: 4g

Raspberry Smoothie

Ingredients:

- 1 cup fresh or frozen raspberries
- 1 banana
- 1 cup almond milk (or any milk of choice)
- 1 tablespoon honey or maple syrup (optional)
- 1/2 teaspoon vanilla extract

Instructions:

1. In a blender, combine the raspberries, banana, almond milk, honey or maple syrup (if using), and vanilla extract.
2. Blend until smooth and creamy.
3. Pour into glasses and serve immediately.

Nutritional Values (per serving):

- Calories: 150
- Fat: 3g
- Carbohydrates: 32g
- Protein: 2g

Watermelon Cubes

Ingredients:

- 1 small seedless watermelon, cut into cubes

Instructions:

1. Cut the watermelon in half and remove the rind.
2. Cut the flesh into cubes.
3. Arrange the watermelon cubes on a serving platter.
4. Serve chilled.

Nutritional Values (per serving):

- Calories: 50
- Fat: 0g
- Carbohydrates: 12g
- Protein: 1g

4

90Day Meal Plan with Adjustments and Tips

Day 1:
- Breakfast: Plain Greek Yogurt with Honey
- Lunch: Simple Quinoa Salad
- Dinner: Lemon Herb Roasted Chicken with Steamed Broccoli and Cauliflower

Adjustment Tips:
- If experiencing mild symptoms, add a soothing herbal tea like chamomile with breakfast.
- For dinner, lightly steam broccoli and cauliflower to make them easier to digest.

Day 2:
- Breakfast: Oatmeal Pancakes
- Lunch: Tuna Salad Stuffed Avocado

- Dinner: Baked Cod with Lemon and Herbs

Adjustment Tips:
- Use gluten free oats if you have gluten sensitivity.
- For lunch, ensure avocado is ripe and soft to avoid digestive stress.

Day 3:
- Breakfast: Tofu Scramble
- Lunch: Fennel and Orange Salad
- Dinner: Shrimp and Rice Pilaf

Adjustment Tips:
- Opt for silken tofu for a softer texture.
- For dinner, ensure shrimp is well-cooked and easy to chew.

Day 4:
- Breakfast: Smooth Cottage Cheese with Blueberries
- Lunch: Zucchini Noodles with Pesto
- Dinner: Roast Turkey with Carrots

Adjustment Tips:
- Choose low fat cottage cheese for a lighter option.
- Slice carrots into thin sticks for easier digestion.

Day 5:
- Breakfast: Almond Butter and Banana on Toast
- Lunch: Vegetable Stir Fry with Tofu
- Dinner: Salmon Patties with Dill Sauce

Adjustment Tips:
- Use whole grain or gluten free toast.
- Cut vegetables into small, manageable pieces for the stir fry.

Day 6:
- Breakfast: Banana Oatmeal Smoothie
- Lunch: Grilled Cheese on Gluten Free Bread
- Dinner: Turkey and Spinach Meatballs with Mashed Sweet Potatoes

Adjustment Tips:
- Blend smoothie until smooth to avoid chunks that can be hard to digest.
- Serve sweet potatoes mashed to a creamy consistency.

Day 7:
- Breakfast: Coconut Rice with Mango
- Lunch: Egg Salad on Sourdough
- Dinner: Pulled Pork with Mashed Potatoes

Adjustment Tips:
- Use ripe, soft mango for the breakfast dish.
- Mash potatoes smoothly and add a bit of broth for easier digestion.

Day 8:
- Breakfast: Polenta with Honey

- Lunch: Baked Beet and Carrot Salad
- Dinner: Baked Tilapia with Olive Tapenade

Adjustment Tips:
- Cook polenta to a creamy consistency.
- Grate beets and carrots finely for the salad.

Day 9:
- Breakfast: Rice Cakes with Avocado Spread
- Lunch: Potato Leek Soup
- Dinner: Chicken and Vegetable Kebabs with Sweet Corn Porridge

Adjustment Tips:
- Ensure rice cakes are soft and avoid hard, crunchy textures.
- Puree potato leek soup for a smooth consistency.

Day 10:
- Breakfast: Herbed Ricotta on Gluten Free Toast
- Lunch: Lentil Soup (without skins)
- Dinner: Risotto with Asparagus

Adjustment Tips:
- Use soft, fresh ricotta cheese.
- Cook lentils until very soft and remove skins.

Day 11:
- Breakfast: Low-FODMAP Muesli
- Lunch: Steamed Vegetable Omelette
- Dinner: Creamy Polenta with Roasted Vegetables

Adjustment Tips:
- Ensure muesli ingredients are finely chopped.
- Steamed vegetables should be tender.

Day 12:

- Breakfast: Apple Cinnamon Porridge
- Lunch: Carrot Ginger Puree
- Dinner: Poached Pear Salad with Grilled Chicken

Adjustment Tips:
- Cook apples until soft in the porridge.
- Puree carrots to a smooth consistency.

Day 13:

- Breakfast: Quinoa Breakfast Bowl
- Lunch: Shrimp and Rice Pilaf
- Dinner: Vegetable Stir Fry with Tofu

Adjustment Tips:
- Rinse quinoa thoroughly before cooking.
- Cut vegetables small for easier digestion.

Day 14:
- Breakfast: Steamed Vegetable Omelette
- Lunch: Fennel and Orange Salad
- Dinner: Baked Salmon with Dill

Adjustment Tips:
- Steam vegetables until soft.
- Use boneless, skinless salmon fillets.

Day 15:
- Breakfast: Egg Custard
- Lunch: Grilled Cheese on Gluten Free Bread
- Dinner: Roast Turkey with Carrots

Adjustment Tips:
- Ensure egg custard is smooth and creamy.
- Thinly slice carrots for easier digestion.

Day 16:
- Breakfast: Pumpkin Porridge
- Lunch: Simple Quinoa Salad
- Dinner: Baked Tilapia with Olive Tapenade

Adjustment Tips:
- Cook pumpkin until very soft.
- Flake tilapia to small pieces before serving.

Day 17:
- Breakfast: Rice Cakes with Avocado Spread
- Lunch: Egg Salad on Sourdough
- Dinner: Chicken and Vegetable Kebabs

Adjustment Tips:
- Use soft, ripe avocados.
- Ensure chicken is well-cooked and tender.

Day 18:
- Breakfast: Herbed Ricotta on Gluten Free Toast
- Lunch: Lentil Soup (without skins)
- Dinner: Lemon Herb Roasted Chicken

Adjustment Tips:

- Use fresh, soft ricotta cheese.
- Cook lentils until very soft and remove skins.

Day 19:

- Breakfast: Low-FODMAP Muesli
- Lunch: Steamed Broccoli and Cauliflower
- Dinner: Shrimp and Rice Pilaf

Adjustment Tips:

- Choose soft, easy to digest ingredients for muesli.
- Ensure shrimp is well-cooked and tender.

Day 20:

- Breakfast: Apple Cinnamon Porridge
- Lunch: Carrot Ginger Puree
- Dinner: Pulled Pork with Mashed Potatoes

Adjustment Tips:

- Cook apples until very soft.
- Puree carrots until smooth.

Day 21:

- Breakfast: Quinoa Breakfast Bowl
- Lunch: Zucchini Noodles with Pesto
- Dinner: Baked Cod with Lemon and Herbs

Adjustment Tips:

- Ensure quinoa is cooked thoroughly.
- Slice zucchini noodles thinly for easier digestion.

Day 22:

- Breakfast: Egg Custard
- Lunch: Potato Leek Soup
- Dinner: Turkey and Spinach Meatballs

Adjustment Tips:

- Make egg custard smooth and creamy.
- Puree soup for a smooth texture.

Day 23:

- Breakfast: Pumpkin Porridge
- Lunch: Simple Quinoa Salad
- Dinner: Creamy Polenta with Roasted Vegetables

Adjustment Tips:

- Cook pumpkin until very soft.
- Ensure polenta is creamy and smooth.

Day 24:
- Breakfast: Rice Cakes with Avocado Spread
- Lunch: Grilled Cheese on Gluten Free Bread
- Dinner: Salmon Patties with Dill Sauce

Adjustment Tips:
- Use soft, ripe avocados.
- Flake salmon patties to small pieces before serving.

Day 25:
- Breakfast: Herbed Ricotta on Gluten Free Toast
- Lunch: Fennel and Orange Salad
- Dinner: Roast Turkey with Carrots

Adjustment Tips:
- Use fresh, soft ricotta cheese.
- Thinly slice carrots for easier digestion.

Day 26:
- Breakfast: Low-FODMAP Muesli
- Lunch: Steamed Broccoli and Cauliflower
- Dinner: Shrimp and Rice Pilaf

Adjustment Tips:
- Choose soft, easy to digest ingredients for muesli.
- Ensure shrimp is well-cooked and tender.

Day 27:
- Breakfast: Apple Cinnamon Porridge
- Lunch: Carrot Ginger Puree
- Dinner: Lemon Herb Roasted Chicken

Adjustment Tips:
- Cook apples until very soft.
- Puree carrots until smooth.

Day 28:
- Breakfast: Quinoa Breakfast Bowl
- Lunch: Lentil Soup (without skins)
- Dinner: Chicken and Vegetable Kebabs

Adjustment Tips:
- Ensure quinoa is cooked thoroughly.
- Remove lentil skins and cook until very soft.

Day 29:
- Breakfast: Egg Custard
- Lunch: Potato Leek Soup
- Dinner: Pulled Pork with Mashed Potatoes

Adjustment Tips:
- Make egg custard smooth and creamy.
- Puree soup for a smooth texture.

Day 30:
- Breakfast: Pumpkin Porridge
- Lunch: Simple Quinoa Salad
- Dinner: Baked Tilapia with Olive Tapenade

Adjustment Tips:
- Cook pumpkin until very soft.
- Flake tilapia to small pieces before serving.

Day 31:
- Breakfast: Plain Greek Yogurt with Honey
- Lunch: Egg Salad on Sourdough
- Dinner: Lemon Herb Roasted Chicken with Steamed Broccoli and Cauliflower

Adjustment Tips:
- If experiencing mild symptoms, add a soothing herbal tea like chamomile with breakfast.

- For dinner, lightly steam broccoli and cauliflower to make them easier to digest.

Day 32:
- Breakfast: Oatmeal Pancakes
- Lunch: Zucchini N
-
- oodles with Pesto
- Dinner: Baked Cod with Lemon and Herbs

Adjustment Tips:
- Use gluten free oats if you have gluten sensitivity.
- For lunch, ensure zucchini is thinly sliced and wellcooked.

Day 33:
- Breakfast: Tofu Scramble
- Lunch: Tuna Salad Stuffed Avocado
- Dinner: Turkey and Spinach Meatballs with Mashed Sweet Potatoes

Adjustment Tips:
- Opt for silken tofu for a softer texture.
- For dinner, mash sweet potatoes smoothly and add a bit of broth for easier digestion.

Day 34:

- Breakfast: Smooth Cottage Cheese with Blueberries
- Lunch: Potato Leek Soup
- Dinner: Salmon Patties with Dill Sauce

Adjustment Tips:
- Choose low fat cottage cheese for a lighter option.
- Puree soup for a smooth texture.

Day 35:
- Breakfast: Almond Butter and Banana on Toast
- Lunch: Simple Quinoa Salad
- Dinner: Creamy Polenta with Roasted Vegetables

Adjustment Tips:
- Use whole grain or gluten free toast.
- Ensure polenta is creamy and smooth.

Day 36:
- Breakfast: Banana Oatmeal Smoothie
- Lunch: Grilled Cheese on Gluten Free Bread
- Dinner: Roast Turkey with Carrots

Adjustment Tips:

- Blend smoothie until smooth to avoid chunks that can be hard to digest.
- Slice carrots thinly for easier digestion.

Day 37:
- Breakfast: Coconut Rice with Mango
- Lunch: Carrot Ginger Puree
- Dinner: Shrimp and Rice Pilaf

Adjustment Tips:
- Use ripe, soft mango for the breakfast dish.
- Puree carrots until smooth.

Day 38:

- Breakfast: Polenta with Honey
- Lunch: Fennel and Orange Salad
- Dinner: Baked Tilapia with Olive Tapenade

Adjustment Tips:
- Cook polenta to a creamy consistency.
- Grate beets and carrots finely for the salad.

Day 39:
- Breakfast: Rice Cakes with Avocado Spread
- Lunch: Lentil Soup (without skins)

- Dinner: Chicken and Vegetable Kebabs with Sweet Corn Porridge

Adjustment Tips:
- Ensure rice cakes are soft and avoid hard, crunchy textures.
- Cook lentils until very soft and remove skins.

Day 40:
- Breakfast: Herbed Ricotta on Gluten Free Toast
- Lunch: Steamed Broccoli and Cauliflower
- Dinner: Pulled Pork with Mashed Potatoes

Adjustment Tips:
- Use fresh, soft ricotta cheese.
- Puree potatoes until very smooth.

Day 41:
- Breakfast: Low-FODMAP Muesli
- Lunch: Vegetable Stir Fry with Tofu
- Dinner: Risotto with Asparagus

Adjustment Tips:
- Choose soft, easy to digest ingredients for muesli.

- Cut vegetables small for easier digestion.

Day 42:
- Breakfast: Apple Cinnamon Porridge
- Lunch: Zucchini Noodles with Pesto
- Dinner: Baked Cod with Lemon and Herbs

Adjustment Tips:
- Cook apples until very soft.
- Slice zucchini noodles thinly for easier digestion.

Day 43:
- Breakfast: Quinoa Breakfast Bowl
- Lunch: Tuna Salad Stuffed Avocado
- Dinner: Lemon Herb Roasted Chicken with Steamed Broccoli and Cauliflower

Adjustment Tips:
- Ensure quinoa is cooked thoroughly.
- Use ripe avocado and ensure chicken is well-cooked.

Day 44:
- Breakfast: Egg Custard

- Lunch: Simple Quinoa Salad
- Dinner: Shrimp and Rice Pilaf

Adjustment Tips:
- Make egg custard smooth and creamy.
- Ensure shrimp is well-cooked and tender.

Day 45:
- Breakfast: Pumpkin Porridge
- Lunch: Grilled Cheese on Gluten Free Bread
- Dinner: Salmon Patties with Dill Sauce

Adjustment Tips:
- Cook pumpkin until very soft.
- Flake salmon patties to small pieces before serving.

Day 46:
- Breakfast: Rice Cakes with Avocado Spread
- Lunch: Potato Leek Soup
- Dinner: Turkey and Spinach Meatballs with Mashed Sweet Potatoes

Adjustment Tips:
- Use soft, ripe avocados.

- Puree soup for a smooth texture.

Day 47:
- Breakfast: Herbed Ricotta on Gluten Free Toast
- Lunch: Carrot Ginger Puree
- Dinner: Roast Turkey with Carrots

Adjustment Tips:
- Use fresh, soft ricotta cheese.
- Sparingly slice carrots for easier digestion.

Day 48:
- Breakfast: Low-FODMAP Muesli
- Lunch: Egg Salad on Sourdough
- Dinner: Creamy Polenta with Roasted Vegetables

Adjustment Tips:
- Choose soft, easy to digest ingredients for muesli.
- Ensure polenta is creamy and smooth.

Day 49:
- Breakfast: Apple Cinnamon Porridge
- Lunch: Vegetable Stir Fry with Tofu
- Dinner: Baked Tilapia with Olive Tapenade

Adjustment Tips:
- Cook apples until very soft.
- Flake tilapia to small pieces before serving.

Day 50:
- Breakfast: Quinoa Breakfast Bowl
- Lunch: Steamed Broccoli and Cauliflower

- Dinner: Chicken and Vegetable Kebabs with Sweet Corn Porridge

Adjustment Tips:
- Ensure quinoa is cooked thoroughly.
- Steam vegetables until very tender.

Day 51:
- Breakfast: Egg Custard
- Lunch: Lentil Soup (without skins)
- Dinner: Pulled Pork with Mashed Potatoes

Adjustment Tips:
- Make egg custard smooth and creamy.
- Puree soup for a smooth texture.

Day 52:
- Breakfast: Pumpkin Porridge
- Lunch: Fennel and Orange Salad
- Dinner: Baked Cod with Lemon and Herbs

Adjustment Tips:
- Cook pumpkin until very soft.
- Slice fennel very thinly.

Day 53:
- Breakfast: Rice Cakes with Avocado Spread
- Lunch: Simple Quinoa Salad
- Dinner: Lemon Herb Roasted Chicken with Steamed Broccoli and Cauliflower

Adjustment Tips:
- Use soft, ripe avocados.
- Lightly steam broccoli and cauliflower to make them easier to digest.

Day 54:
- Breakfast: Herbed Ricotta on Gluten Free Toast
- Lunch: Potato Leek Soup
- Dinner: Salmon Patties with Dill Sauce

Adjustment Tips:

- Use fresh, soft ricotta cheese.
- Puree soup for a smooth texture.

Day 55:
- Breakfast: Low-FODMAP Muesli
- Lunch: Tuna Salad Stuffed Avocado
- Dinner: Turkey and Spinach Meatballs with Mashed Sweet Potatoes

Adjustment Tips:
- Choose soft, easy to digest ingredients for muesli.
- Mash sweet potatoes smoothly and add a bit of broth for easier digestion.

Day 56:
- Breakfast: Apple Cinnamon Porridge
- Lunch: Grilled Cheese on Gluten Free Bread
- Dinner: Shrimp and Rice Pilaf

Adjustment Tips:
Cook apples until very soft.
Ensure shrimp is well-cooked and tender.

Day 57:
Breakfast: Quinoa Breakfast Bowl
Lunch: Carrot Ginger Puree
Dinner: Roast Turkey with Carrots

Adjustment Tips:

Ensure quinoa is cooked thoroughly.
Puree carrots until smooth.

Day 58:

- Breakfast: Egg Custard
- Lunch: Vegetable Stir Fry with Tofu
- Dinner: Creamy Polenta with Roasted Vegetables

Adjustment Tips:
- Make egg custard smooth and creamy.
- Cut vegetables small for easier digestion.

Day 59:
- Breakfast: Pumpkin Porridge
- Lunch: Egg Salad on Sourdough
- Dinner: Baked Tilapia with Olive Tapenade

Adjustment Tips:
- Cook pumpkin until very soft.
- Flake tilapia to small pieces before serving.

Day 60:
- Breakfast: Rice Cakes with Avocado Spread
- Lunch: Zucchini Noodles with Pesto
- Dinner: Chicken and Vegetable Kebabs with Sweet Corn Porridge

Adjustment Tips:
- Use soft, ripe avocados.

- Slice zucchini noodles thinly for easier digestion.

Day 61:
- Breakfast: Plain Greek Yogurt with Honey
- Lunch: Zucchini Noodles with Pesto
- Dinner: Lemon Herb Roasted Chicken with Steamed Broccoli and Cauliflower

Adjustment Tips:
- If experiencing mild symptoms, add a soothing herbal tea like chamomile with breakfast.
- Lightly steam broccoli and cauliflower to make them easier to digest.

Day 62:
- Breakfast: Oatmeal Pancakes
- Lunch: Simple Quinoa Salad
- Dinner: Baked Cod with Lemon and Herbs

Adjustment Tips:
- Use gluten free oats if you have gluten sensitivity.
- For lunch, ensure zucchini is thinly sliced and well-cooked.

Day 63:
- Breakfast: Tofu Scramble

- Lunch: Tuna Salad Stuffed Avocado
- Dinner: Turkey and Spinach Meatballs with Mashed Sweet Potatoes

Adjustment Tips:
- Opt for silken tofu for a softer texture.
- For dinner, mash sweet potatoes smoothly and add a bit of broth for easier digestion.

Day 64:
- Breakfast: Smooth Cottage Cheese with Blueberries
- Lunch: Potato Leek Soup
- Dinner: Salmon Patties with Dill Sauce

Adjustment Tips:
- Choose low fat cottage cheese for a lighter option.
- Puree soup for a smooth texture.

Day 65:
- Breakfast: Almond Butter and Banana on Toast
- Lunch: Simple Quinoa Salad
- Dinner: Creamy Polenta with Roasted Vegetables

Adjustment Tips:
- Use whole grain or gluten free toast.
- Ensure polenta is creamy and smooth.

Day 66:
- Breakfast: Banana Oatmeal Smoothie
- Lunch: Grilled Cheese on Gluten Free Bread
- Dinner: Roast Turkey with Carrots

Adjustment Tips:
- Blend smoothie until smooth to avoid chunks that can be hard to digest.
- Slice carrots thinly for easier digestion.

Day 67:
- Breakfast: Coconut Rice with Mango
- Lunch: Carrot Ginger Puree
- Dinner: Shrimp and Rice Pilaf

Adjustment Tips:
- Use ripe, soft mango for the breakfast dish.
- Puree carrots until smooth.

Day 68:

- Breakfast: Polenta with Honey
- Lunch: Fennel and Orange Salad
- Dinner: Baked Tilapia with Olive Tapenade

Adjustment Tips:
- Cook polenta to a creamy consistency.
- Grate beets and carrots finely for the salad.

Day 69:
- Breakfast: Rice Cakes with Avocado Spread
- Lunch: Lentil Soup (without skins)
- Dinner: Chicken and Vegetable Kebabs with Sweet Corn Porridge

Adjustment Tips:
- Ensure rice cakes are soft and avoid hard, crunchy textures.
- Cook lentils until very soft and remove skins.

Day 70:
- Breakfast: Herbed Ricotta on Gluten Free Toast
- Lunch: Steamed Broccoli and Cauliflower

- Dinner: Pulled Pork with Mashed Potatoes

Adjustment Tips:
- Use fresh, soft ricotta cheese.
- Puree potatoes until very smooth.

Day 71:
- Breakfast: Low-FODMAP Muesli
- Lunch: Egg Salad on Sourdough
- Dinner: Risotto with Asparagus

Adjustment Tips:
- Choose soft, easy to digest ingredients for muesli.
- Cook asparagus until very tender.

Day 72:
- Breakfast: Apple Cinnamon Porridge
- Lunch: Zucchini Noodles with Pesto
- Dinner: Baked Cod with Lemon and Herbs

Adjustment Tips:
- Cook apples until very soft.

- Slice zucchini noodles thinly for easier digestion.

Day 73:
- Breakfast: Quinoa Breakfast Bowl
- Lunch: Tuna Salad Stuffed Avocado
- Dinner: Lemon Herb Roasted Chicken with Steamed Broccoli and Cauliflower

Adjustment Tips:

- Ensure quinoa is cooked thoroughly.
- Use ripe avocado and ensure chicken is well-cooked.

Day 74:
- Breakfast: Egg Custard
- Lunch: Simple Quinoa Salad
- Dinner: Shrimp and Rice Pilaf

Adjustment Tips:
- Make egg custard smooth and creamy.
- Ensure shrimp is well-cooked and tender.

Day 75:
- Breakfast: Pumpkin Porridge
- Lunch: Grilled Cheese on Gluten Free Bread
- Dinner: Salmon Patties with Dill Sauce

Adjustment Tips:
- Cook pumpkin until very soft.
- Flake salmon patties to small pieces before serving.

Day 76:
- Breakfast: Rice Cakes with Avocado Spread
- Lunch: Potato Leek Soup
- Dinner: Turkey and Spinach Meatballs with Mashed Sweet Potatoes

Adjustment Tips:
- Use soft, ripe avocados.
- Puree soup for a smooth texture.

Day 77:
- Breakfast: Herbed Ricotta on Gluten Free Toast
- Lunch: Carrot Ginger Puree
- Dinner: Roast Turkey with Carrots

Adjustment Tips:
- Use fresh, soft ricotta cheese.
- Thinly slice carrots for easier digestion.

Day 78:

- Breakfast: Low-FODMAP Muesli
- Lunch: Egg Salad on Sourdough
- Dinner: Creamy Polenta with Roasted Vegetables

Adjustment Tips:
- Choose soft, easy to digest ingredients for muesli.
- Ensure polenta is creamy and smooth.

Day 79:
- Breakfast: Apple Cinnamon Porridge
- Lunch: Vegetable Stir Fry with Tofu
- Dinner: Baked Tilapia with Olive Tapenade

Adjustment Tips:
- Cook apples until very soft.
- Flake tilapia to small pieces before serving.

Day 80:
- Breakfast: Quinoa Breakfast Bowl
- Lunch: Steamed Broccoli and Cauliflower
- Dinner: Chicken and Vegetable Kebabs with Sweet Corn Porridge

Adjustment Tips:

- Ensure quinoa is cooked thoroughly.
- Steam vegetables until very tender.

Day 81:
- Breakfast: Egg Custard
- Lunch: Lentil Soup (without skins)
- Dinner: Pulled Pork with Mashed Potatoes

Adjustment Tips:
- Make egg custard smooth and creamy.
- Puree soup for a smooth texture.

Day 82:
- Breakfast: Pumpkin Porridge
- Lunch: Fennel and Orange Salad
- Dinner: Baked Cod with Lemon and Herbs

Adjustment Tips:
- Cook pumpkin until very soft.
- Slice fennel very thinly.

Day 83:
- Breakfast: Rice Cakes with Avocado Spread
- Lunch: Simple Quinoa Salad
- Dinner: Lemon Herb Roasted Chicken with Steamed Broccoli and Cauliflower

Adjustment Tips:

- Use soft, ripe avocados.
- Lightly steam broccoli and cauliflower to make them easier to digest.

Day 84:

- Breakfast: Herbed Ricotta on Gluten Free Toast
- Lunch: Potato Leek Soup
- Dinner: Salmon Patties with Dill Sauce

Adjustment Tips:

- Use fresh, soft ricotta cheese.
- Puree soup for a smooth texture.

Day 85:

- Breakfast: Low-FODMAP Muesli
- Lunch: Tuna Salad Stuffed Avocado
- Dinner: Turkey and Spinach Meatballs with Mashed Sweet Potatoes

Adjustment Tips:

- Choose soft, easy to digest ingredients for muesli.
- Mash sweet potatoes smoothly and add a bit of broth for easier digestion.

Day 86:

- Breakfast: Apple Cinnamon Porridge
- Lunch: Grilled Cheese on Gluten Free Bread
- Dinner: Shrimp and Rice Pilaf

Adjustment Tips:

- Cook apples until very soft.
- Ensure shrimp is well-cooked and tender.

Day 87:

- Breakfast: Quinoa Breakfast Bowl
- Lunch: Carrot Ginger Puree
- Dinner: Roast Turkey with Carrots

Adjustment Tips:

- Ensure quinoa is cooked thoroughly.
- Puree carrots until smooth.

Day 88:

- Breakfast: Egg Custard
- Lunch: Vegetable Stir Fry with Tofu
- Dinner: Creamy Polenta with Roasted Vegetables

Adjustment Tips:

- Make egg custard smooth and creamy.
- Cut vegetables small for easier digestion.

Day 89:
- Breakfast: Pumpkin Porridge
- Lunch: Egg Salad on Sourdough
- Dinner: Baked Tilapia with Olive Tapenade

Adjustment Tips:
- Cook pumpkin until very soft.

- Flake tilapia to small pieces before serving.

Day 90:
- Breakfast: Rice Cakes with Avocado Spread
- Lunch: Zucchini Noodles with Pesto
- Dinner: Chicken and Vegetable Kebabs with Sweet Corn Porridge

Adjustment Tips:
- Use soft, ripe avocados.
- Slice zucchini noodles thinly for easier digestion.

5

SUPPLEMENT GUIDE

Supplements in Diverticulitis Management

Diverticulitis, a condition characterized by inflammation and infection of the diverticula in the digestive tract, often requires comprehensive management strategies. Supplements, in addition to traditional therapies like antibiotics and dietary changes, can be extremely important in promoting gut health and reducing symptoms. This article examines many supplements that could help people with diverticulitis.

Fiber Supplements

Role in Diverticulitis: Fiber is paramount in preventing constipation, a risk factor for the development of diverticulitis. By normalizing bowel movements, fiber helps reduce pressure in the colon and the risk of diverticula formation.

Types and Usage: Soluble fiber supplements such as psyllium husk can be particularly beneficial. It is important to increase fiber intake gradually and ensure adequate hydration to prevent bloating and gas.

Probiotics

Role in Diverticulitis: Probiotics support the maintenance and restoration of a balanced population of gut bacteria, which might be upset by diverticulitis episodes. They may help reduce inflammation and prevent infections.

Types and Usage: Supplements containing Lactobacillus and Bifidobacterium strains are often recommended. Taking probiotics during and after treatment with antibiotics can help replenish beneficial gut bacteria.

Turmeric

Role in Diverticulitis: Turmeric contains curcumin, a compound with strong anti-inflammatory properties. It can help reduce inflammation associated with diverticulitis and promote healing.

Types and Usage: Curcumin supplements are available, though absorption can be enhanced with piperine, a compound found in black pepper.

Aloe Vera

Role in Diverticulitis: Aloe vera is known for its soothing properties on the digestive tract. It can help calm irritation and inflammation in the gut, providing relief from symptoms.

Types and Usage: Aloe vera juice or supplements can be used, but it is crucial to choose products free from aloin, which can be harsh on the gut.

Omega-3 Fatty Acids

Role in Diverticulitis: Omega-3 fatty acids, found in fish oil, have potent anti-inflammatory effects that can help reduce the inflammation of diverticulitis.

Types and Usage: High-quality fish oil supplements or algae-based omega-3 supplements are beneficial. It's important to check for purity and absence of heavy metals in these supplements.

Ginger

Role in Diverticulitis: Ginger has anti-inflammatory and antioxidative properties, helping to manage inflammation and protect the gut lining.

Types and Usage: Ginger can be consumed in the form of capsules, teas, or raw in smoothies.

Slippery Elm

Role in Diverticulitis: Slippery elm has a mucilage content that can help soothe the mucous membranes of the gut, reducing irritation and aiding in the healing process.

Types and Usage: It is typically taken as a powder mixed with water or as capsules.

Precautions and Consultation

Before include any supplements in your diet, especially if you're attempting to cure a medical condition like diverticulitis, it's imperative that you contact a doctor. In order to prevent any side effects or interactions, they can provide advice based on your particular medical needs and the medications you're taking.

By integrating these supplements under professional guidance, individuals with diverticulitis can potentially see improvements in their gut health and overall symptom management, enhancing their quality of life.

Essential Supplements for Gut Health

Since the stomach affects everything from digestion to the immune system, maintaining gut health is crucial for overall health. Here are some essential supplements that can support gut health:

Probiotics

Benefits: Probiotics help maintain a healthy balance of gut bacteria, essential for proper digestion, absorption of nutrients, and immune function. They can also reduce the prevalence of harmful bacteria and help in conditions like irritable bowel syndrome (IBS) and inflammatory bowel disease (IBD).

Common Strains: Lactobacillus, Bifidobacterium, and Saccharomyces boulardii.

Prebiotics

Benefits: Prebiotics are fibers that the body cannot digest. They serve as food for probiotics, promoting the growth of beneficial gut bacteria. This maintains a healthy gut microbiota, aiding digestion and increasing immunological function.

Sources: Supplements often contain inulin, fructo oligosaccharides (FOS), and galacto oligosaccharides (GOS).

Digestive Enzymes

Benefits: These supplements help break down food components like fats, proteins, and carbohydrates, aiding in the absorption of nutrients. They are particularly useful for people with enzyme deficiencies, pancreatitis, or digestive disorders.

Types: Amylase (starch digestion), lipase (fat digestion), and protease (protein digestion).

Fiber

Benefits: Fiber supplements can help regulate bowel movements and prevent constipation. They also aid in weight management, help control blood sugar levels, and reduce cholesterol.

Types: Soluble fiber (such as psyllium husk) and insoluble fiber (such as wheat bran).

Omega-3 Fatty Acids

Benefits: As anti-inflammatory fatty acids, omega-3s can help lessen intestinal inflammation, which is advantageous for diseases including Crohn's disease and ulcerative colitis.

Sources: Fish oil and algae-based supplements.

Glutamine

Benefits: This amino acid is a major fuel source for the cells of the intestine. It promotes gut health by aiding in the repair and growth of intestinal cells and may help some gut conditions like leaky gut syndrome.

Usage: Available in powder or capsule form.

Collagen Peptides

Benefits: Collagen helps support and strengthen the protective lining of the digestive tract. This can be beneficial for preventing leaky gut and other intestinal issues.

Sources: Hydrolyzed collagen supplements, which are easily digested and absorbed.

Turmeric (Curcumin)

Benefits: Curcumin, the key ingredient in turmeric, has strong anti-inflammatory qualities that may help reduce discomfort and inflammation in the gastrointestinal tract.

Usage: Often taken with piperine (found in black pepper) to enhance absorption.

Aloe Vera

Benefits: Aloe vera can soothe and calm the digestive tract, helping to relieve symptoms of IBS and other inflammatory gut conditions.

Form: Available as juice or capsules, it's important to choose products free from laxative components like aloin.

Licorice Root (DGL)

Benefits: Deglycyrrhizinated licorice (DGL) helps soothe gastrointestinal issues by coating and repairing the stomach lining and reducing acid reflux.

Form: Available in chewable tablets or capsules.

Before beginning any supplement regimen for gut health, it is essential to see a healthcare provider to ensure that the recommendations are suitable for your particular needs and that there are no adverse drug interactions or health concerns.

Anti-Inflammatory Supplements

For individuals suffering from diverticulitis, managing inflammation is crucial. Several supplements known for their anti-inflammatory properties can be particularly beneficial:

Omega-3 Fatty Acids are recognized for their powerful anti-inflammatory effects, crucial for patients dealing with diverticulitis. They aid in gastrointestinal tract inflammation reduction, which is especially advantageous during flare-ups.Fish oil supplements, which include the potent forms of omega-3s EPA and DHA that are directly linked to the inflammatory response, are the most popular source of omega-3s.

Turmeric (Curcumin) contains curcumin, a compound with significant anti-inflammatory properties. Curcumin helps modulate the body's inflammatory processes through its effects on various biological pathways involved in inflammation. It's often recommended to take turmeric with black pepper (which contains piperine) to enhance its absorption and effectiveness.

Ginger contains active compounds like gingerols that offer strong anti-inflammatory benefits. Ginger is a useful supplement for managing diverticulitis since it can help relax the digestive tract and reduce inflammation.

Due to its anti-inflammatory qualities, Indian frankincense, or Boswellia serrata, has been utilized in traditional medicine. It functions by preventing the body from producing specific inflammatory chemicals, which helps lessen intestinal discomfort and swelling during diverticulitis episodes.

Well-known for its calming effects, aloe vera helps ease digestive system tension and relieve diverticulitis-related inflammation. It is crucial to utilize aloe vera supplements that are made especially for internal use and devoid of aloin, a substance that might irritate the digestive tract.

Licorice Root (Deglycyrrhizinated Licorice or DGL) is a form of licorice that does not contain glycyrrhizin, so it doesn't cause the side effects of standard licorice, such as hypertension. DGL lowers inflammation in the gastrointestinal tract and shields the stomach lining, both of which are advantageous for those with diverticulitis symptoms.

Although silymarin, or milk thistle, is best recognized for its liver-protective qualities, it also possesses anti-inflammatory qualities that may help with digestive issues. The active component, silymarin, relieves symptoms by assisting in the reduction of intestinal tract inflammation.

Consult a physician before using anti-inflammatory supplements to be sure they are suitable for your particular situation and to steer clear of any possible drug interactions. These supplements can be an important component of a more comprehensive diverticulitis therapy plan, assisting in the reduction of inflammation and ease of suffering.

Supplements to Aid Digestion

A number of supplements are made expressly to facilitate digestion and may be quite beneficial for those who are having problems with their digestive system or who wish to enhance their digestive health in general. These supplements maintain the health of the gastrointestinal system and improve nutrition absorption and breakdown in various ways.

These supplements work in different ways to enhance the breakdown and absorption of nutrients and to support the health of the gastrointestinal tract.

Digestive Enzymes contain enzymes that mimic the natural enzymes produced by the body. They help break down fats, proteins, and carbohydrates, making it easier for the body to absorb nutrients. Common enzymes include lipase for fats, protease for proteins, and amylase for carbohydrates. They are particularly beneficial for people with enzyme deficiencies or conditions such as pancreatitis and cystic fibrosis.

Probiotics are good microorganisms that live in the digestive system. For the immune system, food absorption, and digestion to function at their best, a healthy gut flora is necessary. Supplements containing probiotics can help keep this equilibrium. They may also inhibit the growth of harmful germs and diminish the symptoms of gastrointestinal disorders including inflammatory bowel disease (IBD) and irritable bowel syndrome (IBS).

Prebiotics are indigestible fibers that feed good microorganisms in the stomach. Prebiotics aid in better digestion and gut health by promoting the development and activity of these bacteria. Foods rich in prebiotics include onions, garlic, bananas, and asparagus, but they can also be taken as supplements.

Betaine Hydrochloride (HCL) can help increase stomach acid levels, which may be beneficial for people with low stomach acid (hypochlorhydria). Sufficient stomach acid is necessary for efficient food digestion and nutrient absorption.

Ginger is known for its anti-inflammatory properties and can also promote digestion by stimulating saliva, bile, and gastric enzymes that aid in breaking down food. It can help alleviate nausea and is beneficial in treating digestive disturbances.

Since peppermint oil relaxes the muscles in the digestive tract, it can help lessen bloating and spasms. This is why it is frequently used to treat IBS symptoms. It is commonly taken in capsule form to avoid heartburn, which can be a side effect when consumed as a tea or in other forms.

One of the main sources of energy for the cells of the small intestine is glutamine. It supports the repair and growth of intestinal lining and can be helpful in conditions like leaky gut syndrome, where the barrier function of the intestine is compromised.

Licorice Root (DGL), or Deglycyrrhizinated licorice, is used to soothe gastrointestinal problems. By enhancing mucus production, DGL helps protect the stomach and esophagus from acid.

Even while taking these supplements can support and enhance digestive health, you should always see a doctor before using them, especially if you are on other medications or have underlying medical conditions. This ensures that the supplements are used safely and effectively, and that they are appropriate for your specific health needs.

Vitamins and Minerals

Minerals and vitamins are essential for preserving overall health, which includes digestive system health. Certain vitamins and minerals are particularly important for supporting the digestive tract and ensuring the body efficiently absorbs nutrients from food.

Vitamin A the integrity of the digestive tract's mucosal linings, which operate as a barrier against dangerous infections, depends on vitamin A. It is also involved in the regeneration of mucosal cells, which is crucial for healing any damage to the gut lining.

Vitamin C not only boosts immunity but also promotes tissue healing, especially in the digestive tract. As an antioxidant, it helps combat inflammation, potentially reducing the inflammatory responses in conditions like diverticulitis.

Vitamin D plays a role in immune function and inflammation regulation. It's increasingly recognized for its benefits in the gastrointestinal tract, where it helps manage the immune responses and maintain the health of the gut lining.

B Vitamins, particularly B12, and folate, are vital for cell production and the repair of tissues in the digestive system. They help maintain the strength and integrity of the gut wall, which can prevent complications such as diverticulitis and ensure proper nutrient absorption.

Zinc is a mineral that is essential for a healthy immune system and the repair of tissue, including the tissues in the gut. A zinc shortage can worsen gastrointestinal problems by impairing wound healing and weakening the immune system.

Magnesium plays a diverse role in the body, including nerve function, regulating muscle contractions, and digestion. It helps the muscles in the digestive tract function properly, which can prevent constipation and ensure regular bowel movements.

Iron is crucial for the production of blood cells and can be particularly important if there's bleeding associated with gastrointestinal disorders. However, it must be taken carefully, as excessive iron can worsen inflammation and lead to further gut issues.

Calcium is not only essential for bone health but also for the proper functioning of the digestive system. It facilitates smooth muscular contractions that carry food through the digestive system by supporting neuronal transmission and muscle activity in the stomach.

A healthy digestive system, tissue regeneration, and improved gut health may all be achieved by ensuring an appropriate intake of these vitamins and minerals. To handle the quantities and combinations of these nutrients, it's crucial to consult with healthcare professionals, especially if you have any specific medical issues or are on other drugs.

Herbal Supplements for Gut Health

Herbal supplements can be an effective addition to support gut health, offering natural ways to enhance digestive function and alleviate symptoms associated with various gastrointestinal issues. Here are several herbs known for their beneficial properties for the digestive system:

Ginger is celebrated for its potent anti-inflammatory and antioxidant properties, making it a go-to remedy for nausea and digestive discomfort. It stimulates digestion by promoting the secretion of digestive enzymes, improving motility, and helping to ease gas and bloating.

Peppermint has a calming impact on the digestive tract's muscles, which may assist with irritable bowel syndrome (IBS) symptoms including gas, bloating, and sporadic stomach discomfort. Because peppermint oil capsules allow the herb to enter the colon directly, they are especially beneficial.

Chamomile is another herb that is commonly used for its calming effects. It can soothe the digestive tract, relieve irritations, and is often used to treat digestive disturbances, including indigestion, gas, and inflammation.

Slippery elm has mucilage, which, when combined with water, forms a slippery gel. This gel is great for treating gastrointestinal system irritation since it covers and calms the lips, throat, stomach, and intestines.

Licorice Root, specifically in its deglycyrrhizinated form (DGL), helps soothe gastrointestinal problems by restoring balance. It's used for indigestion, stomach ulcers, and heartburn by increasing the mucous coating in the intestinal tract, which can protect against stomach acid and other irritants.

Aloe Vera is well-known for its ability to cure the digestive system as well as the skin. Aloe vera juice can aid with disorders like IBS by reducing inflammation, healing the lining of the stomach and intestines, and soothing the lining.

Fennel seeds are used in traditional medicine to help with bloating and are a common remedy for indigestion. Fennel relaxes the gastrointestinal tract's smooth muscles, helping to relieve gas and bloating.

Milk Thistle, known primarily for its liver-protecting effects, also benefits the digestive organs. Silymarin, the active ingredient, can support the liver in detoxifying, which indirectly benefits gut health and is especially helpful for those suffering from indigestion caused by liver issues.

These herbal supplements can provide significant relief and aid in maintaining a healthy digestive system. Before starting any new supplement regimen, it's imperative to see a healthcare expert to ensure safety and proper consumption. This is especially important for those who already have medical conditions or are pregnant or breastfeeding.

Safety and Side Effects

When considering the use of supplements for any health purpose, including digestive health, it is crucial to understand potential side effects and safety considerations. Supplements can offer significant benefits, but they also come with risks, especially when not used appropriately.

Interaction with Medications: A lot of supplements have the potential to either increase or decrease the effects of prescription drugs. For instance, St. John's Wort may lessen the effectiveness of some antidepressants, while blood thinners may be affected by vitamin K supplements. See a doctor before starting any new supplement, particularly if you are using medication.

Overdose and Toxicity: Vitamins and minerals can be toxic at high levels. Fat-soluble vitamins such as Vitamins A, D, E, and K can accumulate in the body, leading to toxicity if taken in excessive amounts. Minerals like iron and zinc can also be harmful in high doses, potentially leading to serious health issues.

Allergic Reactions: Allergies may arise with certain supplements, particularly those that come from plants, fish, or shellfish. From minor rashes to severe anaphylaxis, symptoms can vary widely. It's important to be aware of any personal or family history of allergies before taking supplements.

Gastrointestinal Issues: Certain supplements, especially those intended to improve digestion, can cause gastrointestinal symptoms such as gas, bloating, constipation, or diarrhea. Fiber supplements need to be taken with adequate water to avoid constipation; meanwhile, magnesium supplements can cause diarrhea if taken in high doses.

Quality and Purity Concerns: There may be problems with purity and quality in the supplement market because it is not as strictly controlled as the pharmaceutical industry. Certain supplements can include impurities or might not contain all of the ingredients specified on the label. Choosing products from reputable manufacturers and those that have been independently tested by organizations like the U.S. Pharmacopeia (USP), Consumer Lab, or NSF International can help ensure quality and safety.

Long-term Use: The long-term use of certain supplements can lead to health issues. For example, long-term use of licorice root can cause hypertension, low potassium levels, and fluid imbalances. Herbal supplements like comfrey and kava can cause liver damage if used extensively over time.

Pregnancy and Breastfeeding: Unless expressly advised by a healthcare professional, many supplements should be avoided while pregnant or nursing. Certain ingredients can be harmful to a developing fetus or nursing infant.

Underlying Health Conditions: For instance, those with autoimmune diseases, cancer, or kidney diseases may experience adverse effects from taking certain vitamins, minerals, or herbs.

To minimize risks and enhance the safety of supplement use:

Before beginning any new supplement regimen, speak with your doctor, especially if you are already on medication or have any underlying medical issues.

As directed by the manufacturer or your healthcare professional, abide by the suggested doses and usage guidelines.

Select high-quality goods from reputable manufacturers to avoid contamination or inaccurate labeling issues.

Keep an eye out for interactions and side effects, and talk to your doctor about them if you have any negative responses.

By taking these precautions, you can safely incorporate supplements into your health regimen and leverage their benefits while minimizing potential risks.

Integrating Supplements into Your Diet

Integrating supplements into your diet effectively and safely requires careful consideration of timing, compatibility with your meals, and overall balance with your nutritional intake. Here's some practical advice on how to incorporate these supplements into your daily routine:

Start with a clear understanding of why you are taking each supplement. Whether it's to address a specific health concern, improve your overall well-being, or fill dietary gaps, knowing the purpose will help you determine the best time and way to take them.

Check the labels for specific instructions, as some supplements are best absorbed when taken with food, while others might be more effective on an empty stomach. For example, absorption of fat-soluble vitamins (A, D, E, and K) is enhanced when taken with a lipid-containing meal. In contrast, iron supplements are best taken on an empty stomach to maximize absorption unless they cause stomach upset, in which case taking them with food may be necessary.

Consider the form of the supplement. Capsules, powders, chewables, and liquids each have their advantages depending on your preference and digestive comfort. For example, if you have trouble swallowing pills, a chewable or liquid vitamin may be a better choice for you.

Integrate supplements into your meal routines for consistency. If you take a multivitamin, make it a part of your breakfast routine. If you're taking probiotics or digestive enzymes, include them during or right before a meal to aid digestion.

Be mindful of interactions between supplements and with foods. Some minerals can compete for absorption, such as calcium and iron, so they should not be taken simultaneously. Similarly, high-fiber meals can interfere with the absorption of certain nutrients, so spacing them out from your supplement intake can be beneficial.

Adjust supplement doses based on your dietary intake. If you're already eating a nutrient-rich diet, you might need a lower dose of certain supplements. Conversely, if your diet is lacking in specific nutrients, like during certain life stages or dietary patterns, increasing supplement intake might be necessary.

Listen to your body and adjust as needed. Supplements can have side effects, and your needs may change over time. Pay attention to how you feel, and consult with a healthcare provider if you have concerns or if you plan to use a particular supplement long-term.

Finally, keep track of your supplement intake and review it regularly with your healthcare provider, especially during health check-ups. This will help ensure that your supplement use remains aligned with your health needs and dietary intake.

By according to these recommendations, you may successfully incorporate supplements into your regular meals and regimen, guaranteeing that they enhance your general health without resulting in any imbalances or adverse consequences.

6

DAILY MENTAL HEALTH TIPS

Establishing a Calming Morning Routine

Establishing a calming morning routine can set a positive tone for the entire day, reducing stress and enhancing mental clarity. Here are some activities that can help create a peaceful and mindful start to your day:

Start by waking up gently to avoid the jolt of a loud alarm. Consider using a wake-up light that simulates sunrise or an alarm with gentle sounds. Giving yourself a few minutes to stretch and breathe deeply before getting out of bed can ease the transition from sleep to wakefulness.

Begin your day by hydrating with a glass of water. Overnight, your body becomes dehydrated, so replenishing fluids first thing in the morning boosts your metabolism and helps flush out toxins.

Engage in meditation or mindful breathing for a few minutes. By keeping your breathing controlled and your attention on the here and now, this exercise helps you center your thoughts and lower your stress levels.

Incorporate light exercises such as gentle stretching, yoga, or a short walk to invigorate your body and mind. Exercise releases endorphins, which uplift the mood and give you more energy, and it also stimulates blood flow. Savor a wholesome breakfast to provide your body and mind with energy for the day. Focus on foods that provide energy without spiking your blood sugar, such as oats, yogurt, fruits, and whole grains.

Spend a few minutes journaling your thoughts, intentions for the day, or things you're grateful for. This can clear your mind of any anxieties and cultivate a positive mindset.

Read or listen to something inspiring, whether it's a book, podcast, or music. Consuming something uplifting can motivate and inspire you for the day ahead.

Take a moment to plan your day by reviewing your tasks. Prioritizing your activities can help manage stress and make your day more manageable.

Try to keep the morning free from digital screens to avoid the stress and distraction that checking emails or social media can bring.

If possible, spend part of your morning outside. Your energy and mood can be enhanced by natural light and fresh air. Even a short time in a garden or park can be beneficial.

By including these exercises in your morning routine, you'll be better equipped to face the day with peace, clarity, and readiness. Adapt these suggestions to fit your lifestyle and preferences, ensuring they provide you with the best start to your day.

Building Resilience Through Mindfulness

Practicing mindfulness helps you build resilience by improving your capacity to handle stress and overcome hardship. The practice of mindfulness, which involves being totally present and involved in the moment without passing judgment, has been shown to considerably increase emotional and psychological resilience. Here are some techniques and practices that can enhance mindfulness and resilience in everyday life:

Regular Meditation: Meditation is at the heart of mindfulness. It entails finding a peaceful place to sit while focusing on your thoughts, noises, breathing, or other body parts. Regular meditation can help increase your awareness and acceptance of the present moment, which enhances resilience.

Focused Breathing: This simple technique involves concentrating on your breath, which can help anchor you in the present moment. Practicing focused breathing daily, even for just a few minutes, can reduce stress and anxiety, helping you to manage difficult situations more effectively.

Body Scan Meditation: This involves analyzing your body mentally to find tight areas and then consciously releasing those areas. The practice helps connect the mind and body, promoting relaxation and awareness, which are essential for resilience.

Mindful Movement: Activities such as yoga, tai chi, or gentle walking can be done mindfully by focusing intently on the movement of your body and the feeling of your feet touching the ground or your muscles stretching. These exercises increase resilience and mental concentration in addition to physical strength and flexibility.

Gratitude Journaling: Keeping a daily journal where you list things you are grateful for can shift your focus from what's problematic to what's positive in your life. This shift can significantly increase your resilience by enhancing your overall perspective on life.

Mindful Listening: Engage in conversations where you focus fully on the other person, listening without planning what you'll say next. This practice can improve your relationships and reduce conflict, contributing to greater emotional resilience.

Nature Walks: Reducing stress and enhancing well-being may be achieved by spending time in nature and going on mindful walks in parks or other natural settings. The practice of being mindful of the sights, sounds, and smells around you during these walks deepens your connection to the present moment.

Mindful Eating: This is giving the act of eating your whole attention, savoring every mouthful, figuring out when you're hungry, and quitting when you're satisfied. Your connection with food and general mindfulness may both be enhanced by this exercise, which will promote improved mental health.

Digital Detox: Taking regular breaks from digital devices can help you become more aware of your surroundings and reduce the stress associated with constant connectivity. Periods of disconnection encourage engagement in the real world, boosting mindfulness and resilience.

Through the integration of these mindfulness techniques into your daily routine, you may improve your capacity to manage daily obstacles and cultivate a more robust and resilient attitude. The secret is to be consistent and to genuinely commit to doing these exercises on a daily basis. With time, they can improve your capacity to deal with life's ups and downs more calmly and easily.

Stress Management Strategies

Managing stress is crucial for maintaining overall health, particularly gut health, as stress can significantly impact digestive function and exacerbate conditions like IBS and gastritis. Here are several effective strategies and exercises to manage stress:

Deep Breathing Exercises: One easy yet effective approach to lower stress is to breathe deeply. The nervous system can be soothed by methods such as diaphragmatic breathing, which involves taking deep breaths into the belly as opposed to shallow ones into the chest. Practicing for a few minutes each day can significantly lower stress levels.

Progressive Muscle Relaxation (PMR): Using this method, various body muscular groups are tensed and subsequently released. This exercise relieves built-up tension in your muscles from stress and increases your awareness of your body's feelings.

Regular Physical Activity: Exercise is a proven stress reliever that helps reduce anxiety and improve mood by releasing endorphins, often referred to as feel-good hormones. Activities like walking, jogging, swimming, or cycling can be particularly effective.

Mindfulness Meditation: Practicing mindfulness involves being fully present in the moment and accepting it without judgment. One may practice mindfulness meditation in a variety of ways, such as by using apps or websites to access guided meditations or by sitting silently and focusing on your breathing, thoughts, and sensations.

Yoga and Tai Chi: To improve both physical and mental health, these activities use breathing techniques, physical postures, and meditation. Both are especially effective in reducing stress, improving mental clarity, and enhancing emotional resilience.

Adequate Sleep: A lack of sleep may make stress worse, and getting enough sleep is crucial for overall health. Stress levels can be lowered by creating a consistent, calming nighttime ritual and setting sleep goals of 7-9 hours each night.

Time Management Techniques: Often, stress arises from feeling overwhelmed with responsibilities. Effective time management can help you break tasks into manageable steps and prioritize them, which can reduce feelings of being overwhelmed.

Social Support: Keeping up a support system of friends and family helps ease stress and offer emotional assistance. Engaging in social activities can distract from stressful thoughts and boost your mood.

Cognitive Behavioral Therapy (CBT): This kind of treatment works well in modifying stress-inducing negative thought patterns. CBT helps identify and challenge stressful thoughts and replace them with more balanced and less distressing ones.

Journaling: Expressing what's going on and letting go of tension may both be therapeutically achieved by writing down your ideas and feelings. It can also help you identify sources of stress and find patterns in your behavior that contribute to stress.

Aromatherapy and Essential Oils: Using scents like lavender, sandalwood, or peppermint can reduce stress and promote relaxation. These can be used with diffusers or added to bathwater for a stress-reducing experience.

By incorporating these techniques into your everyday routine, you may successfully manage stress, which will benefit your gut health and general well-being. It's helpful to experiment with several methods to see which ones perform best.

The Role of Good Sleep in Mental Health

Quality sleep is foundational to good mental health. It allows the brain to process the events of the day, consolidate memories, and rejuvenate both the mind and body. Inadequate sleep can exacerbate mood disorders, including anxiety and depression, as well as cause irritability, tension, and diminished cognitive performance. In contrast, consistent, quality sleep can enhance problem-solving skills and emotional resilience, making it easier to cope with daily challenges.

During sleep, the brain cycles through different stages, including deep sleep and REM (rapid eye movement) sleep, both of which are crucial for cognitive and emotional function. Deep sleep helps to restore the body and brain, promoting physical recovery and growth, while REM sleep is important for processing emotions and memories. A lack of adequate sleep can disrupt these processes, leading to decreased emotional and mental resilience.

To improve sleep quality and ensure the brain and body are well-rested, establishing a regular sleep routine is vital. Maintaining a regular sleep schedule, which includes weekends as well, might enhance sleep quality by assisting the body's internal clock. The mind and body can also be ready for sleep by establishing a nightly ritual that encourages relaxation, such as reading a book, having a warm bath, or doing relaxation exercises.

The setting in which one sleeps has a big impact on how well one sleeps. The brain can get signals to wind down from a quiet, chilly, and dark environment. Purchasing a comfortable mattress and pillows can help enhance the quality of your sleep because physical pain can cause sleep disturbances.

Reducing screen time before bed is another useful tactic for enhancing sleep. The hormone that controls sleep-wake cycles, melatonin, may be produced less effectively when exposed to blue light from devices like computers, phones, and tablets. In the hours leading up to bedtime, avoiding coffee and large meals can also assist in avoiding sleep disruptions.

Maintaining a sleep journal might be beneficial if sleep issues are persistent in order to monitor sleep patterns and potential sleep-influencing habits. Healthcare professionals may find this material helpful in diagnosing sleep problems and suggesting the best courses of action.

By prioritizing good sleep hygiene and making necessary adjustments to sleep habits, individuals can significantly enhance their mental health, improving their overall quality of life.

Scan the QR Code and access your 3 bonuses in digital format

🔥 **Bonus 1: SUPPLEMENT GUIDE**

🔥 **Bonus 2: DAILY MENTAL HEALTH TIPS**

🔥 **Bonus 3: 90Day Meal Plan with Adjustments and Tips**

Made in United States
Troutdale, OR
11/21/2024

25133863R00080